CHOCOHOLIC
Diet Book

Sally Ann Voak

BLAKE

Published by Blake Paperbacks Ltd,
98-100 Great North Road, London N2 0NL, England

First published in Great Britain in 1992

ISBN 1 85782 002 9

British Library Cataloguing-in-Publication Data: A catalogue
record for this book is available from the British Library.

Typeset by BMD Graphics, Hemel Hempstead

Printed by Cox and Wyman, Reading, Berkshire

Home Economist Glynis McGuinness
Edited by Georgina Evans
Cover design by Graeme Andrew
Cover illustration and 'after' pictures
of our successful slimmers by Steve Lewis

1 3 5 7 9 10 8 6 4 2

CONTENTS

Foreword		v
1	What is a Chocoholic?	1
2	Chocolate and History	11
3	Reward, Comfort and Guilt	19
4	Overweight Chocoholics – The Big Six	27
5	Chocs Away?	40
6	The Chocoholic Diet – Six Plans That Really Work	46
7	Our Success Stories	72
8	Massage, Meditation and Exercise	94
9	How to Stay Slim and Eat Chocolate	105
10	Choc Full of Taste!	117

The Chocoholic's Food Diary	136
Calorie Guide to Your Favourite Chocs	140
Counselling Groups	154

To Jan and the Chocoholics of Bexleyheath, Kent, who proved
that it is possible to slim *and* sin!

FOREWORD

By Dr. Gaston L. S. Pawan, D.Sc. (Lond), FRCPath.
Consultant in Human Metabolism and Nutrition

Many, perhaps the majority, of overweight persons in the UK and Western Europe are addicted to chocolate, so-called chocoholics, and regularly consume large amounts of this confectionery. However the psychological and dietary complications associated with this addiction are usually overlooked or only given cursory attention by slimmers as well as their health advisors. Failure to deal adequately with this addiction is one of the main reasons why successful slimming is almost unknown among chocoholics.

In this book Sally Ann Voak has drawn on her wide experience over some twenty years as an international journalist, author, broadcaster, and counsellor on health and beauty to thousands of slimmers, to produce this important and comprehensive account of chocolate addictions, the difficulties they cause for slimmers, and sensible methods of dealing with these problems to ensure lasting slimming success.

The author has provided a fascinating account of the origin and historical development of chocolate manufacture, nutritional data on chocolate varieties, and a delightful section on the reputed effects (sexual, legendary and scientific) of chocolate consumption. Simple methods of diagnosing the different types of chocoholics are described, and diets including recipes and menus, based on healthy eating principles to deal with these, are given.

There is a valuable chapter on massage, meditation and exercise which is of benefit to everyone, and a series of case histories of different chocoholics is provided which illustrates the difficulties, and how to achieve success in slimming.

This book will be of enormous help to all overweight individuals wishing to slim. The practical advice, based on the principles of healthy eating, proper exercise and correct mental attitude given in this book, is recommended to everyone interested in attaining a slim figure, good health and physical fitness.

Dr Gaston Pawan is Hon. Senior Lecturer, formerly Senior Lecturer in Metabolism, Department of Medicine, The Middlesex Hospital and Medical School, London. He is Past Chairman of The Board of Studies in Nutrition and Food Science, University of London.

CHAPTER ONE

WHAT IS A CHOCOHOLIC?

The word 'chocoholic' trips smoothly off the tongue... just like the creamy peppermint filling of a dark, crunchy after-dinner mint. But what does the term really mean?

Chocoholism is often mentioned in advertisements to promote confectionery and is used glibly by reed-thin models who might eat a bar of chocolate once a week. People take alcoholism seriously but chocoholism is just an amusing term to describe weak-willed people who can't resist the occasional 'pig-out' on chocolate. If this is true, why are so many people unable to control their insatiable craving for it and why do they long to reduce their chocolate intake?

Frankly, for millions of serious chocolate addicts, there is nothing amusing about chocoholism. Just like the addiction to any drug (and chocolate could almost be described as a 'drug' for it contains chemicals which can affect the body and brain), chocolate addiction takes over your life. The few moments of pleasure you enjoy as you eat that bagful of chocolate truffles, milky bar, or tube of chocolate-covered caramels are quickly forgotten as you pay the awful price – guilt, self-disgust and an overwhelming desire for another 'fix'. Chocolate can become as irresistible as sex, as habit-forming as smoking, and as difficult to give up as both.

What's more, eating too much chocolate makes most addicts put on weight. Chocolate is one of the most fattening 'treats' ever invented because it contains sugar and fat and is high in calories. Eating too much of it has a disturbing effect on the body's blood sugar levels, so cutting down or giving up becomes very difficult indeed. So anyone with a weight problem who is a chocoholic will find it twice as difficult if they try to shed their excess pounds. It is a bit like being on a roller-coaster ride – you are 'high' one minute, 'low' the next and hungry all the time.

In this book, I have set out to prove that it is possible to break that vicious circle and lose weight. What's more, you can even learn to eat chocolate in moderation and enjoy every mouthful.

How do I know? I spent four months working with a group of chocoholics who have all managed to conquer their addiction. Yes, surprising as it may seem, even a severe chocolate binger whose daily 'fix' included six Galaxy bars and two packets of chocolate digestive biscuits, can now enjoy a couple of chocolate Jaffa cakes each day without suffering severe guilt pangs. What's more, she has lost 20lb. Her name is Wendi Cook and she tells me:

'It is unbelievable. I can now go into a confectionery shop, buy just one bar of chocolate, take it home and eat it. Before, I would have to buy two or three bars at a time. I'd eat them in secret, get a short 'fix' which was far from satisfying, then hate myself afterwards. I even hid the chocolates in my children's toy cupboard. My weight was out of control, too. Now, after just four months on the Chocoholic Diet, I have lost weight and feel in control of my life. It's wonderful.'

She did it – so can you. In this book, I'll tell you how. Go on, eat a piece of chocolate now. Enjoy it and don't feel guilty about it. Soon, you will be slimmer, fitter, and in control of those cravings.

HOW THE CHOCOHOLIC DIET WAS CREATED

Most diets are dreamed up by experts who know what's good for us and then try to make us eat it. They impose a set of eating and drinking rules on a group of volunteers and then make their guinea-pigs stick to them. Not surprisingly, the volunteers lose weight because they are highly motivated to do so. We rarely hear about what happens to them when they finish their slimming programme.

I work the other way around. I talk to people first, find out what their problems are, food and drink likes and dislikes and make my slimming advice fit in with them. Sometimes, my own theories turn out to be correct. Sometimes, not. In the latter case, the diets, behaviour and psychological advice I give is modfied to suit the individual or group of individuals who are helping in the experiment. This does not mean that I recommend people to carry on eating junk food and drinking alcohol if that is what has caused their weight problems. But I certainly would not expect them to give up burgers and beer for life! The diets that don't work, are the ones that people can't stick to because they are too finicky, faddish, or just plain impractical.

I also prefer to help people who, for one reason or another, find it very difficult indeed to lose weight. In fact, if they are convinced they can't lose weight, so much the better! In the famous Fatfield Diet experiment, featured in the BBC-TV programme 'Bazaar' and in *The Sun* newspaper, I worked with a group of big-eating, food-loving villagers from the North East of England, who didn't hesitate to tell me what they thought. Together, we evolved a diet plan which advises slimmers to eat huge meals. It worked and is still working. Our Fatfield group is now 60 strong, and growing. To date, the Fatfield slimmers have lost over a half a ton of weight between them.

Several of our Fatfield villagers were chocoholics and I found that helping them to overcome their cravings involved special care, diet plans and counselling. There is no such thing as a simple weight problem, but chocoholics seemed to me to have far more than their fair share of difficulties. Often, they had emotional problems which prevented them from tackling their weight in a satisfactory manner. Some were lonely, shy or felt unloved, even if they seemed to come from a happy family background. In some cases, the stress of daily living was a contributory factor to their weight problems. So, we set up a smaller, separate group of chocolate addicts, all with different kinds of chocolate addiction and all overweight, to dig more deeply into their problems.

All our volunteers were asked to fill in a rigorous questionnaire to find out more about their chocolate addiction. In one-to-one sessions, each slimmer was questioned further about their chocolate likes and dislikes and given a diet plan to follow. As you will find out later in this book, there was no question of giving everyone the same diet. Every chocoholic is different, although they do seem to fall into roughly six 'types', which will be explained in Chapter Four.

As the experiment progressed, the diet plans were modified, introducing more exciting dishes and recipes. Each volunteer was counselled once a week and encouraged to give us plenty of 'feed-back' on progress – or otherwise! In fact, I was surprised and delighted at the way in which the group responded to our counselling sessions. All of them had been subconsciously punishing themselves for being hooked on chocolate and they expected me to punish them too, with harsh words or impatience. Some had been used to this kind of response by slimming-club leaders during previous attempts to lose weight. However, one of the main rules for all overweight people, not just chocoholics, is that guilt is always counter-productive. So, making people feel guilty, or punishing them in any way at all is virtually guaranteed to result in the pounds piling on!

Below, is a quiz based on the questionnaire we sent out to our volunteers. Try it, and find out if you are a true chocoholic!

HOW TO TELL IF YOU ARE A CHOCOHOLIC

As you have bought this book, there is a very strong chance that you are a chocoholic. Perhaps seeing it on the bookstall made you finally admit to yourself that you do have a problem. Here is a very simple quiz to help you find out for sure. Just answer 'Yes' or 'No' to the 20 questions below, then check your score.

1. Are you eating chocolate while you are doing this quiz?
Yes / No

2. Did you buy *The Chocolate Diet Book* because you are worried about your chocolate cravings? Yes / No

3. Did your mum or dad give you chocolate as a reward or comforting treat when you were a child? Yes / No

4. Have you ever hidden a secret hoard of chocolate in a drawer, cupboard, under the bed or in some other hideaway?
Yes / No

5. Do you frequently buy chocolate when you set out to shop for other things – i.e. at the supermarket checkout or garage? Yes / No

6. Have you ever sneaked into the loo at work or at home for a chocolate 'fix'? Yes / No

7. Does your closest relative know how much chocolate you eat? Yes / No

8. Do you eat chocolate after a row with your partner?
Yes / No

9. Do you always choose the chocolate gateau or mousse on restaurant dessert trolleys? Yes / No

10. Do you ever eat more than one bar of chocolate or a whole box of chocolates or packet of biscuits at one sitting?
Yes / No

11. Would you rather eat something chocolate than a proper meal? Yes / No

12. Do you crave chocolate when you see it advertised on television or in magazines? Yes / No

13. Does eating chocolate make you feel more loved and loving? Yes / No

14. Do all your friends buy you chocolates because they know how much you adore them? Yes / No

15. Have you ever started a crash diet before Christmas or Easter so you can eat more chocolate over the holiday?
Yes / No

16. Does eating chocolate seem to give you extra energy?
Yes / No

17. Do you normally eat chocolate alone rather than with other people? Yes / No

18. Do you think your consumption of chocolate is responsible for your weight problems? Yes / No

19. Have you tried to control your lust for chocolate and failed? Yes / No

20. Imagine you are marooned on a desert island with just a grass skirt, a Bounty Bar and some chocolate coins. The natives have offered you a boat in return for your chocs. Would you trade? Yes / No

HOW DID YOU SCORE?

Give yourself one point for every 'Yes' answer, with the exception of question 7. Give yourself a point for answering 'No' to that question.

Less than 5 points? You are a serious chocolate lover who is not yet a chocoholic. However, you are already treading on dangerous ground. For a start, you have yet to learn how to control your consumption of chocolate properly. Do you eat it because you like it, or in response to pressure, or because you crave chocolate for its comfort value? Reading this book will help you find out. If you have a weight problem, you can certainly try one of the diet plans in Chapter Six.

Between 5 and 15 points? Yes, you are a chocoholic. You must sort out your problems now – before it becomes a dangerous addiction. Chocolate is beginning to take over your life, so now is the time to break this pattern for good. Your chocoholism is making you sneaky, moody, unhappy and fatter than you should be. The good news is that you have already taken the first step towards beating it. Well done!

Over 15 points? Wow! You are seriously addicted to chocolate. Thank goodness you bought this book. Read it carefully and follow all our advice. There is a list of counsellors and groups on page 154, who will be able to give you extra help. Please don't be nervous about seeking it. Your chocoholism is very serious indeed. Do write to me at the address on page 154, and let me know how you get on with the diet.

WHAT'S IN CHOCOLATE?

The cocoa bean contains 50 per cent fat, 20-25 per cent carbohydrate, 5 per cent water, 1.5 per cent theobromine, tyramine and 3.5 per cent minerals and vitamins. These include potassium, calcium, iron, magnesium, sodium, phospherous, Vitamin A, thiamine, Riboflavin and niacin.

It also contains a powerful chemical called phenylethylamine, which is found in the human brain. This is a natural amphetamine which is activated when we are in love giving that wonderful 'out of this world' feeling of euphoria.

When cocoa is made into chocolate, a lot of sugar is added – around two-fifths of its weight. Milk chocolate contains even more sugar, plus milk solids. When this sugar gets into your bloodstream it gives you an instant 'high'. This triggers the pancreas into releasing large amounts of insulin to deal with the rise in blood sugar. Unfortunately, ten minutes or so later, your blood sugar level drops dramatically, producing a 'low' and a craving for more.

Chocolate also contains a small amount of caffeine. Although there is far more in a cup of tea or coffee, if you have a chocolate binge you are likely to experience some effects from the caffeine such as flushed cheeks and palpitations.

TEN REASONS WHY CHOCOLATE MAKES YOU FAT

1. Chocolate is the ultimate comfort food. Parents offer it to their children to cheer them up. So, later on we offer it to ourselves when things go wrong. That's why you rush into a sweetshop for a Snickers or a Mars bar when you've had a row with the boss. That's also the reason why you dig into the choccy biscuit tin when you're watching a weepie movie on TV, or have to reprimand your kids for bad behaviour.

2. It is mega-high in calories. If lettuce was as comforting and delicious as chocolate, very few people would have a weight problem. But lettuce contains only 3 calories an ounce, whereas even just a small (2oz/50g) bar of dark chocolate will 'cost' about 250 calories. Since most women put on weight on more than 2000 calories daily, chocolate is dangerous. You only need a couple of bars daily, plus your normal diet, to push your weight up... and up!

3. Chocs are not filling. Your body feels cheated when you replace a proper, balanced meal with chocolate. So, it

responds by craving more! Chocolate contains sugar and fat. Unfortunately, unless it is the nutty kind, it contains no fibre, which is the stuff that makes your tummy feel full and send 'satisfied' messages to your brain. So, unless you are physically sick, it's hard to tell when you have had enough.

4. You can eat chocolate anywhere. It is sociably acceptable to stuff your face with chocolate in the street, at a party, at your desk, on a train. It is less messy to munch a Crunchie bar than a sandwich while you wait for a bus. It is easier to stash away a pack of m&m's than a tub of healthy cottage cheese in your handbag.

5. It is so available! You cannot leave the safety of your own home without being assailed by chocolates – they're shouting 'buy me, eat me' wherever you go – in the garage, in the supermarket, in vending machines, you name it. It's unfair!

6. Chocolate gives you a 'high' as I explained above. This happens when the chemicals, theobromine and tyramine, which chocolate contains are combined with refined sugar. But this is followed by a fall in your blood sugar which makes you immediately crave another 'fix', and this can rapidly become a binge. This effect is intensified if you combine chocolate with caffeine, so cola and coffee drinkers are even more likely to binge.

7. Chocolate can be a substitute for sex. Sounds far-fetched? In fact, chocolate contains a chemical called phenylethylamine which the brain produces when we are in love. This explains why slimmers who have troubled love lives often get choccy cravings. If your weight problems are related to your sex life (and they often are), eating chocolate will make things worse.

8. Advertisements promote chocolate as an exciting treat. A beautiful girl, dressed only in hideously expensive underwear, sits at a window. Sensuously, she bites into a phallic-shaped bar of chocolate and gazes out into the mist. She is obviously waiting for a handsome bloke to arrive and the chocolate is

helping her get into a sexy mood... Cor! If you are trying to cope with two difficult kids, tidy up last night's mess, answer the telephone and do the ironing all at the same time, the idea of a bar of chocolate becomes very appealing indeed. Two bars would be even nicer...and so it goes on!

9. Premenstrual food cravings often include chocolate. Just when women are pacticularly vulnerable, before their monthly period, chocs appear most attractive. With hormones going haywire, causing fluid retention and mood swings, chocolate seems like a soothing drug. Sadly, it just makes things worse.

10. There are no taboos about eating chocolate. Although you may be ashamed of your chocolate addiction, society doesn't frown on you for eating it. If you sat in the pub drinking gin all day, people would talk. But sitting at home stuffing Mars bars is okay. It isn't though, is it?

CHAPTER TWO

CHOCOLATE
AND HISTORY

When you consider chocolate's sensual taste and exotic background it isn't surprising that it is considered such a treat. For centuries, only the very rich could afford it and most of them couldn't eat – or drink – enough to have to worry about its fattening powers. These days, it is available to everyone and costs relatively little compared with other luxury foods.

The ancient Aztecs were the very first chocoholics. They grew the first cacao trees in the Amazon basin in about AD600, and preferred to grind the beans, mix them with chilli powder and serve the resulting brew topped up with water as a frothy drink called Chocolatl. In 1519, the famous Aztec Emperor Moctezuma (Montezuma) entertained the Spanish explorer Hernando Cortés with a banquet which included 50 large jugs of Chocolatl, served up in pure gold cups. When Cortés returned to Spain (after killing poor Moctezuma and conquering Mexico), he took some cocoa beans with him.

At first, the Spanish were not very impressed by the taste of Chocolatl prepared the Aztec way. It gave them severe tummy ache (known later as Montezuma's Revenge!) and was very bitter and unpalatable. However, when sugar and vanilla beans were also brought back from the New World, they were added to the ground-up cocoa beans to make a more palatable drink which they found very acceptable.

For about 100 years, the Spanish had a monopoly of the chocolate trade. Meanwhile, cocoa beans were used as currency in Central America, which meant that most people could not afford to drink chocolate. Ten beans would buy you a rabbit, and a woman for the night, and for a mere 100 beans you could purchase a reasonably fit slave, so choccy 'money' was obviously far too precious to waste.

At the beginning of the fifteenth century, chocolate was introduced in Italy and France and became highly fashionable. Princess Maria-Thérèse of Spain adored it so much that she persuaded her husband, King Louis XIV of France, to try it. He became hooked too and the royal couple had a special 'chocolate-making' maid to prepare it.

Although chocolate was thought to have restorative powers, it must have caused quite a few spreading waistlines among the super rich, for it was very high indeed in fat. The cocoa bean is about 50 per cent fat, so when the drink was made, this would rise to the surface. Some could be spooned off but the majority remained. When the first chocolate house opened in London in 1657, the drink was so fatty that flour, oatmeal or arrowroot was added to counteract this. But, in 1828, a Dutchman named Coenraad Van Houten developed a hydraulic press which removed most of the cocoa butter, leaving behind cocoa powder.

This invention paved the way for Englishmen John Cadbury and Joseph Fry to start producing chocolate bars by blending the ground-up beans with sugar and additional cocoa butter. From the mid-1860s onwards, eating chocolate became more and more popular, and the types of chocolate available became more elaborate. Fancy chocolate assortments began to be sold in beautiful containers, including velvet-covered mirrored caskets and hand-painted boxes. The French and Swiss became masters of the exotic chocolate gift, but it was not too long before the English manufacturers caught up and they in turn were closely followed by the Americans.

It is interesting that many of the first great chocolate manufacturers were also great philanthropists too. Joseph Fry, Henry Rowntree and John Cadbury were all Quakers, attracted to chocolate because, like tea and coffee, it is non-alcoholic. They cared for their workers, providing free medical check-ups, uniforms and even exercise sessions. In France, chocolatier Jean Menier built the first 'chocolate village' for his workers, and, in 1879, George and Richard Cadbury, sons of John, followed suit with the famous village of Bournville, near Birmingham. Today, their newest plant can wrap 15,000 bars of chocolate every hour. In America, Milton Hershey built a model town called Hersheyville, where the famous Hershey bar was developed as a high-energy food for soldiers during World War II.

CHOCOLATE AND EASTER

The craze for eating chocolate Easter eggs made chocolate production become an even bigger money-making industry. Eggs had always been associated with Easter; they are a symbol of fertility, which ties in naturally with the festival of Spring. When the church in Europe adopted the pagan festival of Easter (or Eostre), some regarded eggs as the symbol of the stone being rolled away from Jesus's tomb. Before chocolate, eggs were either painted real ones, or made from anything from precious stones to cardboard.

The French and German chocolate-makers attempted the first chocolate eggs, painstakingly painting individual moulds with paste chocolate. The first British eggs were made in 1875, when Cadbury found a method of making chocolate flow into the moulds. Now, the basic shell shape (which is usually the least calorific part of the egg as it is very thin) is often a container for everything from toys to more choc-bars.

For chocoholics, the Easter festival is nothing short of a fat-making nightmare. Lured into supermarkets and sweetshops by the sight of dozens of beautiful, delicious eggs, chocoholics can hardly be expected to resist them. Sitting innocently on the shelf, those eggs give out a powerful combination of sex, fertility, and irrestible chemical power. No wonder we are almost compelled to buy them. The best way to deal with this temptation, is to be aware of the calorie content of the chocolates and eggs you buy (*see* the guide on page 140), and to go for the lower-calorie sort, and be very determined to eat just one egg, instead of a dozen. The popular Cadbury's Creme Egg is always a good choice, as it contains just 175 calories and is very satisfying in every way!

SEX, LUST AND CHOC-EROTICA

So, is chocolate an aphrodisiac? The early choc-lovers certainly thought so. After all, they had never tried anything remotely like it before. It came from an exotic country, was expensive, sensual-tasting, and had the added advantage of making you feel loved and loving. (Of course, they did not know about phenylethylamine, the chemical that fools the brain into making chocolate-eaters think they are in love, but that did not stop them from experiencing those loving urges!).

They had also heard the legends about the incredible potency of chocolate as a love-making potion: Moctezuma apparently drank vast quantities of it before visiting his wives and instructed his cocoa planters to have sexual intercourse on top of the young growing plants to speed up their growth! Wow! Casanova was also convinced about the aphrodisiac powers of chocolate. He thought that giving his conquests a draught of hot chocolate was a better bet than plying them with champagne which, although it got them in the mood for love, left them feeling too tired and emotional for vigorous action. Today, chocolates are often the very first gift presented to a woman by a new lover or by an old one who fears that love has gone off the boil. Subconsciously, he is hoping that they will inflame his beloved to heights of passion. It may work, but unfortunately too many gifts like that could make his beloved too fat to fondle! The idea of being given a box of chocs is so delicious that very few women can refuse the offer. Even if your man is unlikely to land by helicopter, scale a cliff, then swim through a swamp to bring you your box of Milk Tray, his heart is obviously in the right place if he bothers to buy one at all. Taking chocolate, or chocolates, to bed when you are lonely is, therefore, a very logical thing for a woman to do, for the comfort and 'lift' of the chocs seems like the perfect substitute for a man. Again, this can be dangerous, as going to bed with a man will help you burn off calories, whereas spending too many nights in bed with only chocolate for company will certainly make you put on pounds.

Women have traditionally used chocolate to perk up their men, too. The famous French courtier Madame du Barry apparently gave it to her lovers if they were feeling a bit droopy. The restorative powers of chocolate were thought to be so effective that a seventeenth-century English gentleman would pop into a chocolate house to sip a large tot before visiting his mistress! Or, the mistress would have a cup of hot chocolate ready in the bedchamber to get the poor chap in the mood. Think about that next time you make your partner a steaming cup of chocolate at the end of a busy day! Monks were banned from drinking it in case their ardours got out of hand, and an article written in *The Spectator* in May 1712 warned readers about 'meddling with chocolates, novels and the like, which I look upon as very dangerous.'

CHOCS THAT SHOCK

Once the manufacturers had discovered how to make

chocolate flow into moulds its production became more sophisticated. Eggs were the first moulded chocolate novelties, but they were followed by a flood of unusual, and sometimes very *risqué*, choccy gifts, particularly from the naughty French chocolatiers. Phallic-shaped chocs, chocolate breasts and bottoms could be obtained 'under the counter', while the normal business of selling eggs, bunnies and fondant-filled chocolates was carried on upstairs. Although all this naughtiness stopped during the war years and the austere 1950s, it came back with a bang in the sexy seventies when phallic chocs were sold at the popular sex shops along with other aids to rapturous love-making. Choc erotica is certainly thriving well in the naughty nineties. Rude chocs can now be bought openly in gift shops and are a big hit at Christmas time. One of the best sellers last year was a 'saucy stocking' containing two breasts, two bottoms and a penis. According to the London-based company who make this saucy item, it was bought mainly by women as a gift for their husbands. Madame du Barry obviously had the right idea!

Even innocent chocolate bars usually have some kind of phallic significance. The 'hard, manly' Yorkie bar is a 'truckin'' good example of this kind of imagery, and was fully exploited when its advertising campaign was planned by Rowntree's. Not only is the guy in charge of a large, powerful lorry, but he is eating a large, hard choc-bar, too. So, he has two penis-substitutes in one commercial! No wonder men wanted the choc-bar and women fancied the trucker. In another TV commercial, the girl who gazes out of the window dreamily as she unwraps her Cadbury's Flake is obviously thinking about something very tasty indeed as she bites into it. If a woman watches this advertisement after a broken love affair she is almost compelled to rush out and buy a Flake.

My conclusion is that, in small doses, chocolate is definitely an aphrodisiac. A delicious nibble, tasted when you are in the right mood, with the right person, could turn you onto thoughts of love with all the accompanying physical feelings... and very nice, too. The problems start when chocolate is eaten in large quantities, as a love substitute. That is when weight problems inevitably follow – which may make you feel depressed, unlovely, and unloving. A case in point is famous chocoholic and television personality, Nina Myscow who says, 'When I lived alone, I frequently woke up in the night with the most awful chocolate cravings. Once, I even drove to an all-night supermarket just to buy a chocolate doughnut... and then ate it before it defrosted! Now, I live with my boyfriend and I still occasionally eat chocolate in bed. These days, though, a little nibble is perfectly satisfying!'

TEN HARD-TO-SWALLOW FACTS ABOUT CHOCS!

1. If all the Crunchies sold in a year were placed end to end, they would stretch from Birmingham to Bangkok and back.

2. If all the Creme Eggs made by Cadbury were stacked one on top of each other, the pile of chocs would be ten times higher than Mount Everest.

3. You could fill 60 double-decker buses with a year's production of Double Deckers.

4. Forty Kit Kats are consumed in the UK every second.

5. The amount of milk used in a year's production of Dairy Milk would fill 14 Olympic-size swimming pools.

6. If all the Wispa bars sold were laid end to end, they would stretch 3.15 times around the world.

7. The money spent on chocs and sweets in half-an-hour would pay for all the tickets to a Madonna concert.

8. The weight of chocolate sold each year in the UK is equivalent to the combined weight of 3000 blue whales.

9. Around £100 per second is spent on chocolates in the UK alone.

10. The world's top consumers of chocolates are the Swiss, eating 21.56lb (9.5kg) per head per annum. Next come the Norwegians (17.4lb/7.9kg), closely followed by the British (16.28lb/7.4kg), then the Belgians (15.2lb/6.9kg), the Dutch (14.96lb/6.8kg), the Germans (14.52lb/6.6kg) and the Irish (14.08lb/6.4kg). The Americans only eat 11.29lb (5.1kg) per head, and the Italians are so full of pasta that they can only manage 3.96lb (1.8kg). However, if you add biscuits, confectionery and chocolates together, the sweet-toothed British come top of the world league table, guzzling an amazing 56lb (25kg) per head annually.

CHAPTER THREE

REWARD, COMFORT AND GUILT

Have you ever felt very low and miserable and longed for the comforting arms of your partner or mum, then eaten some chocolate instead? Most people have done exactly the same thing. In fact, there are very powerful reasons why this emotional response to chocolate occurs.

Our love of sweet foods, including chocolate, is strongly associated with childhood and mother love. The very first food a baby tastes is milk, which, like chocolate, has a high fat content. As it grows and tries different foods, a child will naturally go for those with the obvious kind of taste – strong things like tomato ketchup, sweets and chocolate. It is only later on, during adolescence, that our taste-buds develop to appreciate more subtle and sophisticated food and drink.

We become so sensitive to smells as well as tastes, that we can differentiate between very similar tastes to an amazing degree. It is nature's way of helping us to 'tune in' to the wide variety of nutrients we need in our diet, and to learn the subtleties of sexuality – the smells and tastes of love. That is why we generally feel a bit childish when we pour a big dollop of tomato sauce on our sausages, or dive into a bag of m&m's. That childish feeling is also comforting because most of us naturally associate good things with that period of our lives – things such as security, warmth, and love. If our parents habitually rewarded us with sweets for good behaviour or gave us sweet foods when we were upset, then that feeling becomes even stronger.

Psychologist Jane Firbank says, 'People don't realise how much we are governed by these primitive feelings. Did you know, for instance, that the reason we take chocolates to people in hospital is because they have returned to a childlike, helpless state and therefore we feel they should be treated like children? This sounds very condescending, but is in fact flattering because we are offering them love, comfort and nurturing along with the chocs!'

Even the man who brings his girlfriend a box of chocolates is giving her motherly messages as well as sexual ones. 'In effect, he is saying, "I will take care of you,"' says Jane. 'He is able to do this without diminishing his own masculinity in any way, simply by giving the chocolates.'

Jewish mothers are renowned for thrusting food at their children as a love-offering but any mother will spend a lot of time nurturing her child with lovingly prepared food. The problems start when a mother forces her child to eat up chocolate puddings instead of chicken soup!

Jane says, 'If taken to extremes, this can be quite a dangerous thing. The mother is almost saying, "eat my food or you reject me". The child's response will probably be to eat up and shut up, but in later life, he or she may be strongly affected by this. A very dominant mum can push an entire family into chocoholism.'

So, what can a chocoholic do about this? Firstly, recognise that these are all very common problems, so you are not the only one who is likely to 'pig-out' as soon as things go wrong. Secondly, if you are overweight, it makes sense to get into better shape, using this book to help. Once you feel better about yourself, get out and about more, enjoy sports and generally have a good time, there will be fewer opportunities for you to become depressed and have to resort to those 'childish longings'! Below is a list of everyday situations which often trigger a choc attack, with some suggestions of alternative methods of dealing with them. Try them.

SWAPS FOR CHOCS

You don't have to deal with every tricky situation in your life by eating something sweet. But, if you have been conditioned by your parents to deal with 'hurt' by putting chocs into your mouth, it is very hard to kick the habit. You can do it – practice makes perfect.

Here's a guide to ten familiar daily problems and your probable choccy response together with some alternative suggestions.

Time 7am

Problem You've overslept – again! Your partner is unsympathetic and there is no time for breakfast.

Choc Response You buy a tube of chocolate caramels at the paper shop and eat them on the bus or train, kidding yourself that you need the instant energy.

Non-Choc Solution Make yourself a healthy salad sandwich the night before, wrap it in foil, and stick it in the fridge. You can eat that on the way to work, instead of the chocs.

Time 11am

Problem Your boss has just summoned you to his office for being late. You feel fed up and bored stiff with your work. The office trolley has just arrived on your floor.

Choc Response Your eyes alight on the Mars Bars on the trolley, and you buy two – wolfing them down so quickly that you feel queasy.

Non-Choc Solution Take a deep breath, apologize to the boss, and make a list of ways you can improve production in your section or jot down some ideas for a new project.

Get stuck into your work so you don't even notice when the trolley comes around.

Time 1pm

Problem Your partner has just telephoned to cancel your lunch-date together because of pressure of work. You are disappointed and wonder if he or she is telling the truth.

Choc Response You go to the canteen and indulge in a massive lunch of burgers and chips with a bar of fruit and nut chocolate for dessert.

Non-Choc Solution Exercise is the best way to let off steam. Go for a brisk walk in the the park first, then have that canteen lunch. Chances are you'll pick a more balanced meal.

Time 4pm

Problem You suddenly remember that you have promised to give a talk to the Parents' Association at your child's school tonight. Sheer terror strikes – you haven't prepared a thing!

Choc Response You dig deep in your desk or locker and find a few of the chocolate biscuits you keep there. You gobble them up.

Non-Choc Solution Take deep breaths to help you relax. You know your subject and have bags of time to write a few ideas down on the journey home, so there's no need to panic.

Time 6pm

Problem Your partner is in a foul mood (work was hectic today) and starts up an old row about the state of the family's finances in general, and your extravagance in particular.

Choc Response You lock yourself in the loo with a stiff gin and a Mars Bar until the tirade is over.

Non-Choc Solution Put on a soothing tape or CD, sit down with your partner and plan the week's budget together.

Time 9pm

Problem Your talk has gone well but now you are landed with a group of boring parents moaning about fund-raising. They are getting on your nerves and you feel yourself being drawn towards the chocolate swiss roll on the refreshment table.

Choc-Response You take three slices and wolf them down with a cup of coffee.

Non-Choc Solution Excuse yourself, politely, from the parents, make your excuses and go home – you have done your bit!

Time 10pm

Problem While you were out, your mother has phoned to ask why you forgot her birthday, yet again. She wants you to ring back as soon as you get home...

Choc-Response You know there is a Black Forest gâteau in the fridge, so you cut a slice and eat it rapidly. Then, you ring your mum and grovel.

Non-Choc Solution You plan to send your mum flowers in the morning. You put on the anwering machine and watch the News on TV while you sip a soothing cup of tea.

Time 10.30pm

Problem You are feeling sexy, your partner is not and won't even give you a cuddle.

Choc-response You creep downstairs for another slice of gâteau and suffer from indigestion all night long. Result: neither of you get a wink of sleep.

Non-Choc Solution You tickle your partner's feet and tell them a silly, sexy joke. Laughter is the best aphrodisiac of the lot and less fattening than chocolate!

WHY YOU FEEL GUILTY WHEN YOU DON'T SHARE CHOCS

Why is it that eating a whole box of chocs alone is such a guilt-making experience? Have you ever watched one of those Natural History programmes on TV, where a whole colony of monkeys is studied in detail? Next time, watch out for the bit where they look at the way monkeys eat. Notice how, in normal feeding, the monkey is happy to find his own food and tuck into it, but when he finds something really special like a tree with some particularly tasty fruit, he shares it with the whole group. Well, we humans feel the same way.

When we are eating normal, everyday food (e.g. tucking into a bowl of cornflakes, or eating lunch in the canteen) there is absolutely no question of sharing our meal. In fact, our family or workmates would be rather taken aback if we did offer them a spoonful of cereal or a second-hand brussels sprout. But, 'luxury' foods like chocolate are very different. Instinctively, we feel that these foods must be shared out and we feel like the biggest meanie in the world if we eat them alone. That's why you feel so furious with yourself if you eat up a whole boxful of chocs. You may even lie about it to your family, using excuses like 'the dog had them', or 'I threw them away by mistake.'

WHY YOU CAN'T RESIST CHOCOLATE PUDDINGS

Imagine that you have been out with friends for a fantastic meal and decided to forget your diet for once. You started with a few drinks and nibbles, then had a substantial starter which was a meal in itself – a huge prawn cocktail, pasta dish, or fat-loaded pâté. Then, along comes the main course – steak, onion rings, chips, peas, plus a side-salad washed down with a few glasses of wine. You feel absolutely stuffed and decide not to have any pud.

Suddenly, the waiter wheels the sweet trolley up to your table, and you get a whiff of chocolate gâteau. Amazingly, your brain is suddenly telling you that your tummy is empty and you need some chocolate gâteau, even though you most certainly don't. You succumb, and tuck into a huge slice.

Why did you do it? Blame nature! We are 'programmed' to eat a variety of foods in order to obtain the many different nutrients we need to keep our bodies ticking over. So, when a powerful new food, smelling and looking absolutely luscious is presented to us after a meal, we can still find room for it. In effect, we are 'stocking up' with the luxury food in case we don't get offered any more for a long time. This is obviously nonsense, since we are very likely to have some more chocs the following day, but our primitive urges are very powerful indeed.

You can beat this, and similar potentially dangerous encounters with chocolate, by with some 'mind over body' exercises. Try these:

1. Before going out for a meal, sit down quietly and imagine yourself eating it. Make sure you have a clear picture in your mind of what will happen after your main course. Picture yourself selecting the fresh fruit salad from the trolley. Keep that image tucked away for later on. You can do it!

2. Before you go to a supermarket, write a list of everything you need. Now picture yourself at the check-out. You walk past the sweet and chocolate counter and you do not put anything in your trolley.

3. Before you go into a fast-food restaurant, imagine yourself choosing a fairly sensible meal of burger, bun and fruit juice. After this meal you are feeling very full and satisfied, and do not want a chocolate shake or slice of gâteau. In your imagination, you can see yourself getting up from the table and leaving the restaurant without succumbing to temptation.

4.   Before you go to a friend's home for dinner, have a clear idea in your mind about the food you will be eating. Try to 'see' yourself sitting at the table, eating a good meal, but refusing the chocolate after-dinner mints because you are just too full up to eat them. Go so far as to practise saying to your hostess, 'No thank you. The rest of the meal was so filling and delicious that I just haven't room for anything else.'

CHAPTER FOUR

OVERWEIGHT CHOCOHOLICS – THE BIG SIX

As you will have learned by reading the first few chapters of this book, there are plenty of good reasons why people become hooked on chocolate. In fact, it's amazing that more people haven't succumbed to the 'disease', particularly in the United Kingdom, where £2.4 billion worth of chocolate is consumed annually. That is about £100 a second, and enough to buy 5000 Rolls Royces, 60 Jumbo jets, or 1000 Gary Linekers!

Despite the recession, this figure is increasing by nearly 3 per cent per annum. Today, we eat over 200 million Cadbury's Creme Eggs every year and enough Dairy Milk to cover all the pitches in the football league. If you've got a taste for this kind of statistic, recheck the list on page 17 when you feel a severe case of choccy cravings coming over you – the images they conjure up could help put you off. (If they don't, you certainly do need this book!)

Since the calories supplied by 1oz (25g) of milk or plain chocolate is approximately 150, it is not surprising that many (although not all) chocoholics have weight problems. Although a mere 150 calories might not sound much, when you consider that the weight of a typical chocolate bar (such as a Galaxy) would be around 3½oz (85g), it means that the total calories consumed in a whole bar would be over 400. A chronic chocoholic would have no trouble at all in putting away over 1000 calories of chocolate daily. If he or she is in a sedentary job and eats a fairly normal diet as well as the chocolate, that exta 1000 calories daily could result in a gradual weight-gain of around 2lb weekly.

At this point let me say that, in my 20 years' experience of working with slimmers, calories do count! Yes, I know that some lucky people can burn energy more quickly than others but the simple fact remains that if you consume fewer calories than you expend you will lose weight. Sorry, folks, it's painful but true. So, never trust a diet that says you can eat as much as you like of foods other than those that are so low in calories (e.g. green vegetables and salads) that you'd have to eat a ton to put on a pound. Certainly never trust a diet that says you can eat anything you like – even for just an hour or so a day. A determined chocoholic could easily stuff 3000 calories worth of chocs in that time without pain (until later!).

A calorie is a unit of energy: the amount that, if converted into heat, would raise the temperature of 1 gram of water by 1 degree Centigrade. This is a very small unit indeed, so when scientists are measuring food intake, they use a unit that is a thousand times larger, called a kilocalorie (kcal for short). However, most slimming writers, including me, don't bother with the kilo prefix. All you really need to know is that the average woman in a sedentary job uses around 2000 calories each day, and the average man will use something between 2500 and 3000 daily.

Some foods are more calorie intensive than others (i.e. they pack a whole lot of calories into a very small mouthful), particularly those high in fat – like cheese (116 calories for just an ounce of Cheddar) or butter (210 calories per oz). Sweet foods are calorie-intensive too. An ounce of white, granulated sugar contains 112 calories, and even a level teaspoon can set you back 20 calories. Chocolate is high in fat and sugar, so it is one of the most calorie-intensive foods you can consume. When I call it a 'food', I mean just that because both fat and sugar are nutrients – although we should eat less of them. Unfortunately, we can't live on fat and sugar alone; we need other foods, such meat, fish and eggs, vegetables, cereals and fruit, to supply all the nutrients that keep us healthy. So, it is not surprising that chocoholics frequently surpass their daily calorie requirements, and therefore put on weight easily. It has been estimated that, next to hard drugs, the three biggest 'crutches' for overstressed humanity are cigarettes, drink and chocolate. What a pity that the least physically harmful of the three is not a low-calorie, full-of-goodness food... then we could all indulge with a clear conscience and a slim waistline!

WHICH CHOC-LOVER ARE YOU?

During our research with chocolate cravers, we found that most sufferers fit into one of six chocoholic 'types', and some span a couple of categories.

Establishing which type of chocoholic you are is the first step towards controlling your chocoholism. That is because each type needs a slightly different version of the basic diet, and also different behavioural and psychological 'exercises' to help break the habits, tensions and thought patterns that are making them fat and miserable.

Below is a guide to the six main categories. At the end of each section you will find a list of questions which you should answer honestly. They will help you decide which diet plan to follow. If your particular problems mean that you fit into two categories, follow the diet plan and 'exercises' which fit in best with your lifestyle and food tastes. (For instance, some women find that they become Premenstrual Cravers just before a period, but need the Comfort Eater diet and lifestyle strategy at other times of the month.)

Before you tackle the questions at the end of each section, read the general information on each type very carefully. As you read, you will start to recognise things about yourself that you may not have acknowledged before. Please, don't feel despondent or 'put down' by this. Remember that acknowledging your fat-making habits and problems is the first step towards doing something about them.

TYPE ONE: SECRET BINGERS

Characteristics The secret binger thinks, sometimes mistakenly, that no one knows about his or her choccy cravings. They sneak into sweet shops out of town to buy their secret supplies of chocs, in the hope that they won't bump into a neighbour or friend. They then hide the stores of chocolate in an unlikely place – a child's toy cupboard, garden shed or airing cupboard – and go back later on to stuff themselves. These binges usually happen when they are tired, emotionally upset, feeling lonely, or desperately hungry (e.g, after a day or two trying to follow a crazy diet).

The last thing a secret binger wants to do is admit they have a problem. So, they usually refuse chocolate in a social situation, generally protesting that they are 'on a diet' or 'can't stand the stuff'. They may even refuse chocolate-flavoured puddings or an after-dinner mint on the grounds that chocolate 'doesn't agree' with them, and then go back home and reach for the supply in their secret hiding place.

A secret binger is adept at finding odd places for binges – such as in the loo or parked in a car in a lonely layby. The sad thing is that the binge is not an enjoyable experience – it produces feelings of guilt and often nausea. If they are unable to conquer their furtive chocolate eating habits, secret bingers can develop very serious problems such as bulimia, and frequently need expert one-to-one or group counselling.
Background The secret binger is often someone who has

been brought up with high expectations of achievement. Weaknesses like over-indulgence in chocolates were probably not tolerated lightly in his or her family. As a child, they may have been expected to do exceptionally well academically or at a sport. They may even have achieved high standards, but never perhaps reached the very top – or maybe they feel that they have passed their 'peak'. Sometimes, the secret binger is someone who is weighed down by family responsibilities and problems – single parents, and those with money worries can fall into this category. Many women become secret chocolate bingers when they are faced with domestic problems like bringing up difficult teenage children who don't get on with their father or step-father. Youngsters who are under pressure to do well in exams and men who have been made redundant from work are also at risk.

QUESTIONS

1. Is there a secret hoard of chocolate hidden somewhere in your office, home, or car?

2. Do you intend to eat it alone?

3. Are you satisfied with what you have achieved in your career and personal relationships?

4. Do you think your parents are (or would be) proud of you?

5. Do you feel that you have to do more than your fair share to keep your family happy?

6. Do you ever feel resentful about the lack of fun, leisure time, or sexual satisfaction in your lifestyle?

7. Have you ever followed a low-calorie diet for a few days, then 'pigged-out' on chocolate?

8. Have you ever refused to eat chocolate when out with friends, then had a private orgy afterwards?

9. Do you feel very guilty indeed about your chocoholic habits?

10. Are you keeping this book well hidden so no one realises that you have got a problem?

If you answered 'yes' to most of the questions except numbers 3 and 4, you are a Secret BInger. Your diet and strategy are on page 48.

TYPE TWO: ROMANTICS

Characteristics Since chocolate has such a powerful effect on the psyche and senses, it is no wonder that it is often used as a love-substitute. The Romantic is a person who is simply not getting the physical and emotional affection and understanding that he or she deserves. So, instead of having a romantic time in bed, a cuddle with a loved one or just a loving conversation, they eat chocolate.

Romantics are often single, unattached and lonely. Or, they can be trapped in a loveless or boring relationship. They often buy expensive and unusual chocolate as a substitute for an expensive and unusual lover. Romantics wake up in the night, usually alone, and fancy an orgy of Mars bars or a quick 'fix' of Kit Kat. Female romantics often go for phallic-shaped choc bars like Toblerone or Cadbury's Flake. Men might choose softer, rounder treats like Cadbury's Creme Eggs or the soft-centred chocs in Quality Street packs.

Background Romantics tend to undervalue themselves as lovers. Maybe they have had a bad experience, or experiences ... or maybe they have never had a lover. If they have been in a stable relationship, it's usually the Romantic who has put all the hard work into it. They feel that chocolate can take over when romance fails. It is more reliable, easily available, reasonably cheap, and you don't need to use a condom to enjoy it! It doesn't matter how successful the Romantic is in his or her career, they feel a failure in love, and somehow unworthy of being loved. Eating chocolate makes them feel sexy and wanted even if it's only for a very short time.

QUESTIONS

1. Do you think you are attractive to the opposite sex?
2. Currently, do you have a caring partner?
3. Do you feel that you get enough cuddles?
4. Do you enjoy choccy treats in the middle of the night?
5. Have you ever consoled yourself with a chocolate eating orgy after a broken romance?
6. Does the smell of chocolate make you feel sexy?
7. Are you particularly fond of expensive Swiss or Belgian chocolate?
8. When you've eaten chocolate, do you feel a sense of satisfaction that is so powerful it is almost sexual?
9. Do you crave less chocolate when your love-life is going smoothly? (Think about it!)
10. Do you make jokes about your choc-loving habits?

If you answered 'no' to questions 1, 2 and 3, but 'yes' to most of the others, then you are a Romantic. Your diet and strategy are on page 61.

TYPE THREE: COMFORT EATERS

Characteristics This is by far the most common type of chocoholic. The Comfort Eater eats chocolate when stressed, lonely, tired, or faced with problems. In acute cases, the sufferer will tuck into chocs all day long, rather than deal with the underlying cause or causes of the cravings. For example, a Comfort Eater may be in a high-pressure job with deadlines to meet. When things get tough, they instinctively turn to the chocolate-vending machine, canteen or trolley. Often, Comfort Eaters live alone – students, divorced and separated people for instance. They tend to buy chocolate on a daily basis, rather than hoarding it. You will see highly stressed Comfort Eaters desperately throwing a few choc bars in their trolley at the supermarket check-out point and probably tucking in to one or two in the car park.

Background Comfort Eaters have usually been given chocolate as a comfort food in childhood, and the habit of eating something sweet and creamy when stressed has stuck. They usually have a pile of problems (possibly no more than other people, but they just seem more), which they find difficult to cope with. There may be no one sympathetic enough to talk to (perhaps partners are unwilling or too busy to help). Because they lack organisation, Comfort Eaters will kid themselves that it is quicker and easier to snack on chocolate than to have a proper meal.

QUESTIONS

1. Did your parents give you chocolate as a 'comfort' food when you were a child?

2. Do you think you are overworked, overstressed, overwrought – or even all three?

3. Do your problems seem to get more complicated every day?

4. Are you ever lonely (even if you are living with someone)?

5. Have you ever eaten a chocolate bar while sobbing your heart out?

6. Do you enjoy eating chocs while you watch weepy movies on TV?

7. If someone gives you chocs, do you mean to eat them gradually but wolf the lot down when you feel the blues coming on?

8. Do you eat chocolate while you are waiting (impatiently!) at bus-stops, stations or queuing at the bank?

9. If the washing machine flooded what would you do first – eat a chocolate biscuit or call the plumber?

10. If your partner throws a wobbly, would you rather go up to your bedroom with a box of chocs than sit down and discuss the situation?

If you answered 'yes' to seven or more of the questions, then you are a Comfort Eater. Your diet plan and strategy are on page 52.

TYPE FOUR: WEEKEND INDULGERS

Characteristics This is the chocoholic who uses every weekend, holiday and outing as an excuse for a sweet treat – or several! Friday night is for stocking up with chocs, from the garage, the supermarket or from the local confectioner's shop on the way home from work. Men tend to favour the garage as a purchasing point for its convenience and macho image. It is fine for a man to buy chocs when he is paying for petrol, too 'feminine' to be seen doing so in a confectionery store or supermarket. The Weekend Indulger will sometimes pretend that this mound of goodies is for 'the kids', but in fact most of it is destined for 'grown-ups'. The Weekend Indulger is also an Easter and Christmas chocolate junkie, even going to the trouble of losing a few pounds before each of these annual eating orgies so they can indulge with a relatively clear conscience. The Weekend Indulger loves chocolate puddings on Sundays (and by way of an excuse explains that this is 'the only day of the week I allow myself to eat them'), chocs for occasions like theatre and cinema outings, and they often give boxes of expensive chocs to other people so they can nibble them too!

Background Again, childhood behaviour patterns are very important, for the Weekend Indulger usually comes from a family where chocs were considered an important part of family celebrations. The Weekend Indulger continues this family tradition with a vengeance, especially when he or she is having a stressful time, or when they may be in an unsatisfactory relationship. They have to learn that they can have fun without necessarily eating chocs too. They also need plenty of oral gratification, so kisses, cuddles and sensual food are all very important.

QUESTIONS

1. Were Easter Eggs and Christmas chocs an important part of your childhood?

2. Do you buy most of your chocs on Fridays or before a holiday or outing?

3. When you go out for a meal, do you feel vaguely disappointed in your evening unless you've enjoyed a choccy dessert from the dessert trolley?

4. After such an evening, are you likely to tuck into a few chocolate biscuits at home before bedtime?

5. Do you ever pretend to buy chocolate for your children, and eat it yourself?

6. Is a trip to the theatre incomplete without a box of chocolates?

7. Do you like to eat chocolate on Sunday afternoon or evening, when you are relaxed and feel that you deserve a treat because it is your day off?

8. Does your partner often bring you chocs as a present?

9. Do you like to eat chocolate slowly, savouring every mouthful?

10. Does the smell and taste of chocolate conjure up happy memories for you?

If you answered 'yes' to seven or more of the questions, you are a Weekend Indulger. Your diet and strategy are on page 64.

TYPE FIVE: SUGAR ADDICTS

Characteristics Sugar Addicts are 'hooked' on sugar, rather like chronic smokers are hooked on nicotine. They obtain most of their daily calories from carbohydrate, using chocolate bars as a 'fix' when they feel tired, hungry, or fed up. Dancers, models, actors, students and even sports people can fall into this category. Dancers, particularly, who are terrified of putting on weight, may stop eating conventional meals, grabbing chocolate bars to fill the energy gap. Unfortunately, sugar addiction can be extremely dangerous, leading to long-term health problems.

Background Pressure is the problem for most Sugar Addicts. They are under pressure to perform, achieve, and keep going, in all circumstances. This pressure may have started back in their childhood or teens, or be self-generated once the Sugar Addict has entered the rat race. The feeling of being on a treadmill is, sadly, increased by their diet. The craving for sugar must be satisfied at all costs (like the craving for a cigarette), but once it has been satisfied, there is only a short respite before another 'fix' is needed. This is because chocolate creates a blood sugar 'high', which is quickly followed by a 'low'. It is a vicious circle of craving which is very hard to break.

QUESTIONS

1. Are you in a job which requires very high standards of mental and physical performance?

2. Are you usually too rushed to stop for breakfast and lunch?

3. Do you ever feel weak and wobbly because you have missed several meals?

4. Are you then likely to eat a chocolate bar or sweet snack rather than make time for a proper meal?

5. Are you generally uninterested in gourmet eating?

6. Do you live alone or share a flat with friends?

8. Do you believe that we need a certain amount of sugar each day to keep going?

9. If someone cut off your chocolate supplies completely, would you worry that you could not do your job properly?

10. Do you keep a chocolate bar, or bars, in your handbag, briefcase or work bag for emergencies?

If you answered 'yes' to seven or more of these questions,

especially numbers 1, 2, 3 and 4, then you are, or are becoming, a Sugar Addict. Your diet and strategy are on page 68.

TYPE SIX: PREMENSTRUAL CRAVERS

Characteristics   Most chocoholic women have fallen into this category at some time or other. Many become Premenstrual Cravers for a few days every month, when they may find themselves stuffing chocolate bars at very strange times indeed – in the bath, at the hairdressers, waiting outside the school for the children, in the middle of an important meeting at work. At this time, they may even buy brands of chocolate which they do not normally fancy.

Background   Hormonal activity just before a menstrual period can cause tension and even severe depression. One theory is that these symptoms are caused by Vitamin B deficiency. Lack of Vitamin B means that the liver cannot break down the monthly build up of the hormone oestrogen. An excess of oestrogen causes an imbalance of chemicals in the brain and it is thought that too many stimulating chemicals are made and not enough dopamine, which normally has a soothing effect on the body. Adequate levels of B vitamins (particularly Vitamin B6) and magnesium are needed for normal dopamine production. Chocolate contains a relatively high level of magnesium, so that terrible craving for chocs could be your body's way of telling you that your stores are low. Unfortunately, the chocolate is so high in sugar, too, that it will definitely make you feel worse. Better by far to take Vitamin B6 and eat more leafy vegetables and cereals!

QUESTIONS:

1.   Do you feel even more frantic to eat chocolate during the week before your monthly period?

2.   Do these cravings strike so fiercely that you have to buy a bar of chocolate immediately, even if it means missing a train or being late for an appointment?

3.   Are you more inclined to eat the chocolate quickly than savour it slowly?

4.   Are you often accused by your family of being extra touchy at this time of the month?

5.   Do you take Vitamin B just before your period?

6.   Do you buy special chocs to cheer yourself up?

7.   Is the week after your period the only time when you can lose weight?

8.   Do you make any extra effort to pamper yourself and relax when you are premenstrual?

9.   When trying to slim, have you always had difficulty in curbing your choc-eating habits at this time of the month?

10.   Do you also sometimes crave more cigarettes and/or alcohol as well as chocolate?

If you answered 'yes' to most of the questions except numbers 5 and 8, then you are a Premenstrual Craver and you should follow the diet and strategy on page 56.

CHAPTER FIVE

CHOCS AWAY?

Imagine being told to eat ten bars of chocolate every day and keep the wrappers piled up on your office desk for everyone to see. That is the kind of treatment that is recommended for chocoholics by some behaviour therapists. Their argument is that this kind of therapy will, eventually, make the sufferer give up. Personally, I am pretty sure that it would make them throw up... but giving up is something else!

Even the shame of knowing that other people are disgusted by their behaviour, is not enough to help severe chocoholics stop. It simply makes them switch to eating chocolate in secret, which can cause all kinds of physical and psychological problems including obesity and depression.

After talking to many, many chocolate 'junkies', I am convinced that it is much more sensible to cut down on your chocolate intake and learn to enjoy it in small quantities. You can only do this by following a good diet plan which is specifically designed to keep your blood sugar level high and to make you feel in great shape.

A chronic sufferer who expanded from a size 12 to a size 22 after becoming hooked on chocolates told me, 'Chocoholism is the same as being an alcoholic but without Alcoholics Anonymous to help. I even tried the Samaritans, who were kind but didn't know much. There's acupuncture, if you can afford it, and doctors aren't much help. Mine recommended anti-depressants!' She recovered after following a vitamin and mineral rich diet for six months, and now sticks to the same basic plan. She has also managed to lose 3 stone in weight and is still losing.

Well-known chocoholics include superstar Cher, Nina Myscow, Lulu, Judge James Pickles and Elizabeth Taylor.

Cher, world-famous singer and actress, loves m&m's and is very partial to Häagen-Dazs chocolate icecream. She is, however, very interested in nutrition and has worked out a diet with her nutritional adviser, Dr. Robert Haas. This diet keeps her blood sugar level high all day so she does not get choccy cravings too often. She also maintains that exercise is a tremendous help. It could well be that the endorphins, a group of chemicals manufactured in the brain, which are produced by rigorous exercise give a similar 'high' to that experienced after a chocolate 'fix'. Exercise is certainly helpful in alleviating stress and maximising energy levels. Cher still has occasional binges which are usually triggered by stress or exhaustion. Her diet and exercise control her chocoholism but will never beat it. During the making of the movie *The Witches of Eastwick*, she admits to having chocolate orgies with fellow actress Michelle Pfeiffer who is also a choc fan.

Nina Myscow has tried all kinds of chocoholic cures. She says, 'My mother used to stuff food in my mouth to shut me up. I graduated from biscuits to doughnuts to the sensual pleasure of chocolate. By the time I reached my thirties, I was an expert. I have gorged myself on bars of Cadbury's Whole Nut and stuffed myself silly with chocolate-covered doughnuts.'

'My worst-ever crisis was when I came home from a holiday in West Africa and bought two huge slabs of chocolate when I changed planes at Geneva Airport. I only meant to eat one on the plane but found myself sitting next to a wizened

Japanese businessman instead of a handsome hunk. I ate both through sheer disappointment and felt even worse.'

'In my time, I have tried crazy crash diets, hypnosis, you name it. But the only thing that works is to eat sensibly, take exercise and learn to enjoy chocolate when you have it. Now, I can eat one perfectly formed white Belgian chocolate each week and relish every mouthful. I can also go into a newsagent and just buy the papers, a can of diet coke and a small pack of nuts and raisins. I wouldn't say that I am cured, but I definitely have the problem well under control.'

The singer, Lulu, inherited her chocoholism from her mum, Betty. 'My mother and I are still so keen on chocs that we would rather have a chocolate snack or pudding than a proper meal. I have beaten it though and I can now limit my chocs to a treat every day. But when mum and I get together we have to be very strong indeed!'

Lulu agrees that there is no such thing as a cure for the affliction and declares that she wouldn't want one. 'I'd hate to think that I could never again sit down to my favourite, French-style breakfast of a croissant with a piece of rich, dark chocolate,' she says. 'So, I now allow for it in my daily diet. I think you've got to look at the whole you when you're trying to improve your life. Take a step back and try and work out what is making you so dependent on chocolate. I've found that meditation helps me in everything from dealing with work problems, to planning what to eat.'

James Pickles, the famous former British judge, loves expensive chocolates. 'I am very partial to Thornton's chocolates', he says, 'and I can easily eat a lot of them. It is even harder now I have retired from the bench because I work at home and it's easier to get hold of chocolate. So my wife Sheila has to hide them from me!' But Judge Pickles is managing to control his cravings and recently lost half a stone on a version of the Chocoholic Diet.

Elizabeth Taylor, the superstar actress, now has her weight under control again after years of 'yo-yo' dieting. Her addiction to junk food and chocs seems over now that she is happily married to Larry Fortensky. She says, 'People say that chocolate tickles the love centres of the brain, so when you are in love you don't need it. Maybe that's what's happened to me!' It is also likely that the sensible and healthy diet she and husband Larry have been following has helped control her urges for chocolate.

Here is a round-up of six ways of controlling chocoholism and the pros and cons of each method:

1. *Quitting 'Cold Turkey'* This method is often used successfully by smokers. They make a New Year's resolution to quit on 1 January and do so – just like that! It only works for smokers if they have prepared themselves mentally for the day when they quit. This includes reading up everything they can lay their hands on about the dangers of smoking, ear-marking the precise items they will buy with the cash they save, and giving themselves other rewards like holidays, outings and luxuries. Problems arise when they hit a stressful situation where they cannot turn to their usual 'prop'. That's why so many former smokers become sweet-oholics instead, put on weight and go right back to smoking again!

Chocolate addiction is just as complex as nicotine addiction, but is related to comfort and guilt as well as stress and physical cravings. Only someone with the most amazing willpower could give up a six-Mars-a-day habit just like that! In fact, if anyone reading this book has been able to do it, I would very much like to hear from them (my address is on page 154).

Trying to give up chocolates completely is quite dangerous because it frequently leads to a very bad binge once the next 'crisis' (whether it's a lover's tiff or something far more serious) occurs. What does work well is to cut out chocolate completely for a week or a couple of weeks, while altering your eating habits. The discipline of doing so gives you a boost, and you still have the promise of chocolate to come at a later date, even though it will be in smaller quantities. Meanwhile, good nutrition is helping you to arm yourself to eat chocolate in moderation. This method worked very well with volunteers who tried out the various programmes on The Chocoholic Diet.

2. *Cutting down* If your body is used to a massive amount of sugar each day, you will probably feel faint and ill for a few days if you try to cut down. Again, the only answer is to change your eating habits at the same time. You must make sure that you eat regularly, and have alternative snack foods available. The diet on page 110 (How to Stay Slim) can help if you are not very overweight, but feel that a healthier diet, and fewer chocs, would be good for you. It will, it will!

3. *Hypnotism and acupuncture* These treatments may help addicts cope with symptoms like depression and guilt but they will not turn a confirmed chocoholic into a choc-hater. You must want to cut down before these can help. One acupuncturist told me, 'I get people with all kinds of cravings asking for treatment, including chocolate cravers. But, acupuncuture is not a cure-all and I can only offer a treatment to supplement nutrition therapy.' A hypnotist who has had terrific success with smokers says, 'Chocoholism is different. I once had a patient who weighed 25 stone and ate three boxes of chocs and ten bars of chocolate every day. She was told by her doctor that she would probably have to be brought into hospital unless she could control her chocolate intake because of complications caused by her weight problems. She had high blood pressure and a heart murmur. The fear of hospitalisation made her want to beat chocoholism, so we worked out a plan which involved a hospital

diet and hypnotism. The hypnotism did help, but I'm sure it was her own fear and the diet which really made her cut down. She was very receptive to my therapy, and that is absolutely essential if it is going to work. So far, she has managed to lose 3 stone, and we are still working well together, but it is a slow process.'

4. *Behaviour therapy* Like hypnotism and acupuncture, behaviour therapy can only be part of a chocoholic's cut-down campaign. However, it is a very useful part. While I would not advise the type of therapy described in the first paragraph of this chapter, I do think that monitoring how, when, and why you eat your chocs is a very helpful. Check through the points listed on pages 136-139 for your own behaviour therapy guide.

5. *Crash dieting* This can help you lose a lot of weight very fast, but you will put it back on again even more rapidly. Once you come off a diet that is below around 1500 calories for men, or 1000 for women, your body is programmed to store any extra calories. As a chocoholic, these calories are likely to be in the form of your favourite high-fat, high-sugar treat. So, you'll end up eating more chocolate, not less.

6. *Exercise* The benefits of exercise are well-documented, but for those who have not experienced them it is worth giving a few reminders here. Exercise can help strengthen your heart, reduce blood pressure, and prevent stress. It can also help you maintain your correct body weight and cut your appetite. The feeling of well-being produced by exercise is an effective substitute for 'props' such as nicotine, alcohol and chocolate. All the chocoholics we worked with while re-searching this book found that regular exercise (a minimum of 20 minutes' aerobic exercise – i.e. swimming, jogging, dancing) helped improve their self-image and made them a whole lot happier. However, exercise alone is unlikely to help overweight chocoholics cure their cravings or lose any weight.

CHAPTER SIX

THE CHOCOHOLIC DIET: SIX PLANS THAT REALLY WORK

Here they are, the six diet plans that can turn chocolate cravers into calm, controlled, slim people

By completing the quiz in Chapter Four, you should already have discovered which kind of chocoholic you are. If you feel that you fall into two categories, try one plan first, and see how it goes. All the plans have one thing in common: they include regular, filling meals that keep your blood sugar level high, so you are *never* hungry.

Our chocoholic volunteers found that learning to eat regularly was the very first step towards conquering their addiction. While you continue to neglect your body by missing meals, snatching empty snacks and following crash diets, you will never cure your chocoholism. Emotional and behavioural triggers that precipitate an attack are hard enough to conquer without the additional burden of acute, tummy-rumbling hunger pangs.

So, please follow your diet faithfully, without missing any meals at all. If you hate eating breakfast, you can pack it up and take it with you to work. Don't be tempted to miss out on that first, vital meal of the day.

THE FIRST WEEK
Please stop eating chocolate altogether for the very first week of your diet. This is important because it is a vital part of

learning to control your cravings. On subsequent weeks, you will be given an allowance of chocolate, chosen from the list on page 140 or the recipes in Chapter Ten.

Clear out any hoards of chocolate which you may have stashed away in the house. Give them to a neighbour, your mother-in-law or throw them away. Make sure there are no hidden chocs in the freezer, in the glove compartment of your car or under the bed. If other members of the family are chocolate eaters, ask them to keep the chocs out of your sight just for the first week of your diet.

FREE VEGETABLE LIST
All six diets allow unlimited amounts of certain, very low-calorie vegetables. Pile them up on your plate but do not add butter or margarine or salad dressings other than lemon juice, vinegar and herbs. It is important that you munch your way through as much as you can of these 'free' veggies – they supply valuable vitamins and minerals which will help you in your fight against chocolate addiction. Here is the list:

asparagus	fennel
beansprouts	gherkins
broccoli	leeks
Brussels sprouts	lettuce
cabbage	mushrooms
cauliflower	mustard and cress
celery	peppers (red and green)
chicory	radishes
Chinese leaves	runner beans
chives	shallots
courgettes	spinach
cucumber	spring onions (scallions)
curly kale	tomatoes (canned or fresh)
endive	watercress

MEN Please add around 300 calories to your diet plan by having 2 extra slices of wholemeal bread with a little low-fat spread or a couple of small rolls plus ½ pint extra beer or lager. If you are tee-total, have a small potato instead. If you are in a 'heavy' job, such as construction work, please add an extra 4oz (100g) meat or fish, or 2oz (50g) low-fat cheese as well.

DIET FOR SECRET BINGERS

DAILY ALLOWANCES ½ pint (275ml) skimmed milk, water and mineral water. Drink lots of water – about 6-8 glasses daily. Try to avoid tea and coffee – no more than 2 weak cups of tea daily. Try herbal tea instead. Take a multi-vitamin capsule every day.

FREE VEGETABLES Eat as much as you like from the 'free' vegetable list. You can boil or steam veggies, or serve them as salads. Do not add butter or margarine, and use lemon juice, vinegar and herb dressings on salads.

CHOCOLATE None the first week, sorry. This is the start of the rest of your life. Once you have your blood sugar level under control, and are psychologically adjusted to living without your chocolate 'crutch', you can gradually re-introduce the chocs. Your allowance for Week Two and subsequent weeks is 150 calories daily (check the chart on page 140 for the calorie count of your favourite chocs).

- Try to halve the amount of cigarettes you normally smoke

- Cut down on alcohol to the amount allowed under Treats

- Do not add salt when cooking. Use herbs, lemon juice and garlic instead.

STRATEGY

1. The act of clearing out your choccy hoards is especially important for you. Starting with a 'clean slate' will help you stick to the diet. You could be surprised at how much this one act of control will help you. Reward yourself afterwards with a good long soak in a scented bath. You can tell someone about it if you like, but don't be surprised or put off if they are less than hopeful about your chances of sticking to the diet – it may be in their interest to keep you fat! Remember, this is for you.

2. Confession time: write down a list of things you are worried about, fear, or are unhappy with in your life. Secret chocoholism is often a sneaky way of avoiding looking at other problems in your life. If you have a good friend (not a relative) who you can discuss this with, do so. Talking it through will help you cope. If you prefer, keep the list private – just writing it is a way of facing things, instead of burying them. Don't forget that you can write to me, at the address on page 154, if you wish. Where problems are very serious, please do seek the help of a trained counsellor. You can get a list at your public library or Citizen's Advice Bureau, or we can help.

3. Treat time: sneaking off for a chocolate binge is now a thing of the past for you ... we hope! Instead, try sneaking off for one of these treats: a facial, massage or manicure; a swim in the local pool; a window-shopping expedition; a walk in the park with a good book for company, and fruit to eat; a browse round a music store.

4. Walk briskly for at least 20 minutes each day. This will help speed up your metabolism, and make you feel less hungry.

5. Go swimming or try some other relaxing exercise once a week – dancing, skating and yoga are also excellent. The exercises in Chapter Eight have been specially devised for chocoholics – try them.

WEEK ONE

EVERY DAY Eat *one* Breakfast, *two* Light Meals, and *one* Main Meal, plus *one* Treat. You can eat them when you like, but please do not leave long gaps between eating. Have a large glass of water before each meal and plenty of water between meals.

BREAKFASTS (200 calories)
- 1 oz any unsweetened cereal, milk from allowance, 1 chopped banana
- Sandwich of 2 thin slices wholemeal bread with 2 tbsp cottage cheese, sliced tomato, a few grapes
- 1 slice wholemeal toast topped with grilled tomatoes, 1 size 3 poached egg
- 1 large slice of melon sprinkled with 2 tbsp cottage cheese, ½oz (12g) mixed nuts, small glass unsweetened orange juice

LIGHT MEALS (250 calories each)
Jacket Potatoes Make a huge salad from the 'free' list (page 47), add 8oz (200g) jacket potato and one of these toppings:
- 2 tbsp baked beans
- ½ carton natural yogurt
- 4oz (100g) carton Shape Coleslaw

Salads Make a huge mixed salad with vegetables from 'free' list (page 47) and serve it with one of these choices:
- 8oz (200g) chicken leg, no skin, grilled or roast, 1 apple or orange
- 4oz (100g) grilled or steamed fish, no sauces, 2 small boiled potatoes, 1 small banana
- 1 small carton cottage cheese, 2 tbsp sweetcorn, 2 chopped apricots, 1 slice wholemeal bread.

Sandwiches 2 slices wholemeal bread with salad from 'free' list (page 47) and one of these fillings:

- 2oz (50g) tuna-in-brine with lemon juice
- 2 tbsp cottage cheese
- 2oz (50g) peeled prawns
- 1oz (25g) lean ham or chicken

Soups
- 1 tin slimmer's soup, any flavour, 1 slice wholemeal bread, 1 carton Diet Ski or Shape Yogurt
- Home-made vegetable soup (use vegetables from 'free' list) with wholemeal croutons, 1 slice toast topped with tomatoes and ½oz (12g) grated Edam cheese

MAIN MEALS (350 calories each) Don't forget to add piles of 'free' vegetables (page 47) and salad.
- 1 large slice of melon, 3oz (75g) canned sardines on 1 slice wholemeal toast, grilled tomatoes, watercress, 1 orange
- 4oz (100g) grilled liver, thin gravy with 2 tbsp fresh orange juice added, 2 small boiled potatoes, 2 tbsp sweetcorn, 1 small banana
- 5oz (125g) lamb chop, thin gravy, 3oz (75g) mashed potato made with milk from allowance, 1 pear or 2 apricots
- Any Findus Lean Cuisine or Heinz Weight Watchers Meal, with 1 piece fresh fruit afterwards
- 5oz (125g) grilled herring or tinned pilchards, 2 small boiled potatoes, 1 serving Bird's Lite Mousse
- 1 well-grilled beefburger, 2 tbsp sweetcorn, 5oz (125g) jacket potato, 4oz (100g) strawberries or raspberries
- 3oz (75g) any lean meat, thin gravy, 2 small chunks roast potato, 1 small wholemeal roll
- 3oz (75g) (cooked weight) wholemeal pasta or wholegrain rice with one of the following toppings and an apple or orange to follow:

- 3oz (75g) prawns with tomatoes, garlic, herbs
- 1oz (25g) chopped ham with tin of slimmer's mushroom soup
- 2oz (50g) chicken breast with tin of slimmer's chicken soup

TREATS (100 calories)   Choose *one* each day.
- 1 glass dry wine
- 2 pub-measure 'short' drinks with low-calorie mixers (use soda or tonic – not sweet-tasting soft drinks)
- ½ pint beer or lager
- 2 crispbreads topped with 2 tbsp cottage cheese, sliced gherkins or 1 tsp sweet pickle
- 1 mug Batchelors Slim a Soup with small slice wholemeal bread

WEEK TWO and subsequent weeks
You may now have 150 calories of chocolate from the Calorie Guide to Your Favourite Chocs on page 140. You may also have *one* 200-calorie dessert or drink from the recipes listed in Chapter Ten (pages 117-135) each day.

DIET FOR COMFORT EATERS
DAILY ALLOWANCES   ½ pint (275ml) skimmed milk for your tea and coffee, unlimited water, mineral water. Please cut down on those cups of tea, substituting herb teas, and more water.

FREE VEGETABLES   You can have as much as you like of the vegetables on the 'free' list (page 47). Serve them lightly boiled or steamed, or as salad. Do not add butter or other fat. Make your own salad dressing using lemon juice, vinegar, black pepper, herbs and garlic. Avoid salt; do not use it in cooking or sprinkle it on your food.

CHOCOLATE 200 calories daily in the second week, decreasing to 150 calories daily in the third week. Buy your chocolate allowance every day, do not hoard it. When you buy it, put it into a tin immediately. Eat your chocolate allowance when things are going well, not when they are going badly. Do not eat chocs when you have had a row with your kids or spouse, nibble them when you are having a jolly time. Choose your chocs from the calorie guide on page 140 or from the recipes in Chapter Ten.

STRATEGY

1. Stress is one of the things that is making you eat more chocolate than you should. You can get the same 'high' from exercise as you do from chocs. While you are following the diet, please attend a health club, gym or aerobics class at least three times weekly. You need the kind of exercise that will make you feel out of breath for around 20 minutes, three times a week. An exercise bike at home can help too. But, cheaper and just as effective, is to run up and down stairs, or use the bottom stair for some 'stepping' exercises.

2. Every day, make a list of all the things you have to do both for work, yourself and your family. As they are accomplished, tick them off. Don't let worries pile on top of you. Try to deal with problems logically. Consult your partner or a friend if you are worried about something. If this is impossible, talk to your doctor or a counsellor. Write to me at the address on page 154, if you need any advice that is not contained in this book.

3. If you live alone or feel lonely even though you live with someone else, it is always a good idea to make contact with organisations in your local community. Doing some charity

work, or joining a club, or going to an evening class will give you a new angle on life. For, even if you are a busy career person (and many chocoholic comfort eaters are high-flyers who boss others around all day), a change is as good as a rest.

4. Talk to someone new every day. That doesn't mean chatting up someone at random, but it means having a pleasant word with someone who's non-threatening like a shop assistant, taxi driver or work colleague who you haven't spoken to before.

5. Try swimming, skating, dancing or a yoga class each week, and do the special exercises in Chapter Eight.

6. When you feel an urge to eat chocs, have a long glass of water, phone a friend, and if you still feel that you must eat a choc, have one of the emergency snacks or treats listed below instead.

WEEK ONE
EVERY DAY Choose *one* Breakfast, *one* Light Meal, *one* Main Meal, and *two* Treats.

BREAKFASTS (200 calories)
- 1 slice wholemeal toast topped with mashed banana and 1 tsp honey
- 1oz (25g) any unsweetened cereal, milk from allowance, 1 apple, two crispbreads with a little low-fat spread
- 1 egg, boiled or poached, 1 slice wholemeal toast
- 4 oz (100g) tinned apricots or figs topped with 1 tsp muesli and 1 tbsp natural yogurt
- 2 tbsp sweetcorn, 3oz (75g) mushrooms poached in chicken stock, grilled tomatoes, 1 grilled vegeburger

LIGHT MEALS (250 calories)
Cooked Meals Any Findus Lean Cuisine or Heinz Weight Watchers Meal of 250 calories (check pack) or under, with a

54

huge pile of vegetables and/or salad from the 'free' list.

Jacket Potatoes   Make a huge salad from 'free' list (page 47), add an 8oz (200g) jacket potato and one of these toppings:

- 2 tbsp baked beans
- ½ carton natural yogurt
- 4oz (100g) carton Shape yogurt

Salads   Make a huge salad using vegetables from 'free' list (page 47), and add one of these:

- 8oz (200g) chicken leg, no skin, grilled or roast, 1 apple or orange
- 4 oz (100g) grilled or steamed fish, 2 small boiled potatoes, 1 small banana
- 1 small carton cottage cheese, 2 tbsp sweetcorn, 2 chopped apricots, 1 slice wholemeal bread

Sandwiches   2 slices of wholemeal bread with salad from 'free' list (page 47) and one of these fillings:

- 2oz (50g) tuna in brine with lemon juice
- 1oz (25g) lean ham or chicken

Soup   Use Heinz Weight Watchers Soups as a base and add extra vegetables from 'free' list (page 47), plus 2oz (50g) chopped chicken, ham, or tuna, 1 small wholemeal roll

MAIN MEALS   (350 calories) Don't forget to add piles of 'free' vegetables (page 47) and salads.

- 3oz (75g) (cooked weight) wholemeal pasta or wholegrain rice with one of the following toppings and an apple or orange to follow:
  - 3oz (75g) prawns with tomatoes, garlic, herbs
  - 1oz (25g) chopped ham with tin of slimmer's mushroom soup
  - 2oz (50g) chicken breast with tin of slimmer's chicken soup
- 1 well-grilled beefburger, 2 tbsp sweetcorn, grilled tomatoes, 1 slice wholemeal bread, 1 large banana

chopped and served topped with a little milk from allowance and ½oz (12g) mixed nuts

- Bird's Eye Menu Master Healthy Options Vegetable or Chicken and Ham Lasagne
- 3oz (75g) any lean roast meat, thin gravy, 2oz (50g) peas, 2oz (50g) carrots, 3oz (75g) chunks roast potato, 1 apple or orange
- 8oz (200g) grilled chicken leg, no skin, 5oz (125g) jacket potato, 1 small banana
- Casserole of 4oz (100g) chicken or fish cooked in 1 tin low-calorie slimmers' soup, with sliced onions and peppers, 3oz (75g) potato, mashed with milk from allowance, 1 carton low-calorie fromage frais
- Takeaway meal of ½ portion medium thin pizza or 1 Kentucky Fried Chicken dinner

TREATS OR EMERGENCY SNACKS (50 calories each)
Choose *one* each day.
- ½ glass dry wine, topped up with soda, and a few grapes
- 2 crispbreads topped with 1 tbsp cottage cheese and chopped gherkin
- 1 small banana
- 10 grapes
- 1 slice Nimble bread topped with salad from 'free' list

WEEK TWO and subsequent weeks
Add 200 calories of chocolate each day decreasing to 150 calories in Week Three and until you reach your goal weight. You may also add *one* 200-calorie dessert or drink from the recipe section each day. But, please make sure you eat it when things are going well!

DIET FOR PREMENSTRUAL CRAVERS

This diet should be followed for one or two weeks before or

during a menstrual period.

DAILY ALLOWANCES ½ pint (275ml) milk for your tea and coffee, unlimited water and mineral water. Try to replace as many cups of tea and coffee as you can with water or herbal teas.

FREE VEGETABLES Eat as much as you like from the 'free' vegetable list (page 47). Do not add butter or low-fat spread, and use just lemon juice, garlic, herbs and vinegar to make a salad dressing.

CHOCOLATE On the second week of your diet, you can have up to 100 calories of chocolate each day from the list on page 140. If you like, save it up for a larger amount, say twice a week. However, if you follow the diet correctly and are not a serious chocoholic you may find that you no longer experience choccy cravings at all.
- During the week before your period, and the week of your period, take two Vitamin B6 capsules and four Evening Primrose Oil capsules each day.
- Do not add salt when cooking. Instead, use herbs, lemon juice and garlic if you like it.

STRATEGY
1. Walk briskly for at least 20 minutes each day. This will help ease tension as well as speed up your metabolism.
2. Do deep breathing exercises in front of your mirror every morning. Start by exhaling slowly through your mouth, then inhale through your nose. Repeat ten times, before facing the problems of the day.
3. Beat tension headaches with exercises for your shoulders and neck: try backwards arm-swings, hunching then relaxing your shoulders, putting your right hand over your right

shoulder and trying to touch it with your left hand, then repeating to the left.

4. Try acupressure: place your middle fingers in the hollow at the side of your head just by your brow bone. Press firmly, hold for a count of six, then relax. This really does help soothe away headaches, so try it before you take a pain-killer; you may not need one.

Have a go at this one too: kneel on a cushion, join your hands together with your fingers-back to back, fingertips pointing towards your tummy. Let your relaxed fingers press into the centre of your tummy, below the ribs, above the navel. Now lean gently forward and exhale. Raise yourself upright as you inhale. Repeat six times, then have a good stretch as you get up. This is a good exercise to help relieve feelings of depression or anxiety.

5. Go swimming once or twice a week or join a yoga or dance class. Swimming is wonderfully relaxing and also exercises every part of your body, but gently. So, it is the perfect sport. Yoga and dance also help beat tension. Don't push yourself into an aerobics class, or go jogging – both can be too exhausting for comfort!

6. When you feel low, give yourself a treat – a scented bath, a walk in the park, a low-calorie lunch with a friend. Don't mope... you can cope!

Now choose *five* 200-calorie meals each day from the lists below, plus *one* treat (including alcohol!). If you like, you can lump a couple of the meals together, but it is best to spread your food allowance out... especially in those dangerous days just before your period.

CEREAL MEALS
- ½ grapefruit, 1oz (25g) any unsweetened cereal topped with a medium banana, milk from allowance

- 1 Weetabix, milk from allowance, 2 crisbreads topped with a little low-fat spread, 1 carton Diet Ski or Shape yogurt
- 1oz (25g) porridge made up with water and milk from allowance, 1 apple, 1 crispbread topped with 1 Kraft Cheese triangle
- 4oz (100g) figs canned in syrup, sprinkled with 1 tbsp unsweetened muesli and topped with 1 carton natural yogurt

FISH MEALS Use 'free' vegetables (page 47) or salad, plus one of the following:
- 4oz (100g) any grilled or steamed fish, 2 small boiled potatoes
- 4½oz (112g) grilled herring, 1 crispbread with low-fat spread
- Findus Lean Cuisine Cod fillet in Tarragon Sauce or Cod Mornay, a few grapes or 2 apricots
- 4oz (100g) any shellfish, 1 slice wholemeal bread

JACKET POTATO MEALS Bake an 8oz (200g) jacket potato, and serve with a huge portion of salad or vegetables from the 'free' list (page 47), plus one of these toppings:
- 2 tbsp cottage cheese or baked beans
- ½oz (12g) grated Edam cheese mixed with tinned tomatoes
- ½ carton natural yogurt with chives

MEAT MEALS Use unlimited 'free' vegetables (page 47), boiled or steamed, with one of the folowing choices:
- 5oz (125g) lean chump chop, with thin gravy
- 8oz (200g) chicken joint, grilled or roast, no skin, thin gravy
- 3oz (75g) any lean roast meat, thin gravy, 1 small boiled potato

- 1 well-grilled beefburger, 1 small (5oz/125g) tin baked
  beans

SALAD MEALS   Make yourself a huge salad using vegetables
from 'free' list (page 47). As well as lettuce and tomatoes, try
raw cauliflower, spinach, cold cooked green beans and
courgettes, etc. Now add one of these choices:
- 3oz (75g) chicken (no skin)
- 2 tbsp sweetcorn, 1 apple
- 4oz (100g) any white fish, grilled or steamed, 2 small
  boiled potatoes
- 7oz (175g) jacket potato, ½oz (12g) grated Edam cheese
- 2oz (50g) lean ham, 1 small wholemeal roll

SANDWICH MEALS   2 thin slices wholemeal bread with
salad from 'free' list (page 47) and one of these:
- 1oz (25g) grated Edam cheese
- 3 tbsp cottage cheese
- 2oz (50g) tuna-in-brine
- 2oz (50g) chicken (no skin)
- 3 tbsp baked beans
- 1 medium banana, chopped with lemon juice

TREATS   (100 calories) Choose *one* of each day.
- 1 glass dry wine
- 2 pub-measure 'short' drinks with low-calorie mixers
- ½ pint beer or lager
- ½oz (12g) unsalted mixed nuts
- 1 large slice wholemeal bread with a little low-fat spread
- 1 large banana
- 1 carton low-calorie fromage frais or yogurt with 1
  medium digestive biscuit

DIET FOR ROMANTICS

DAILY ALLOWANCES   Water and mineral water. ½ pint (275ml) skimmed milk for your tea and coffee.

FREE VEGETABLES   Eat as much as you like from the 'free' vegetable list given (page 47). Do not add butter or low-fat spread, and use just lemon juice, garlic, herbs and vinegar mixed together for a salad dressing.

CHOCOLATE   After the first, non-choc week, you are in for a treat. For, three times weekly, you may 'spend' 300 calories on chocolate. This is a *lot*. Select your chocs from the list on page 140 or the recipes in Chapter Ten. Make sure that you shop no more, and no less, than three times a week. Enjoy the occasion and do not feel guilty about it.

STRATEGY

1. Make a list of all the good things about you – physical, intellectual, everything. Keep it somewhere handy and carry on reading it!

2. Make another list of things that normally 'trigger' a chocolate-craving attack. Study it carefully and see if there is any way in which you can avoid these things, or face them differently.

3. During the diet you must have a personal treat every single day. This can be anything that gives you pleasure – from an hour with a favourite magazine, to a long, scented bath or an evening in with a weepy video. And, yes, you may eat chocolate while you indulge – as long as it is from your allowance (*see* above).

4. If you feel an uncontrollable urge to splurge on chocs coming on, deal with it by (a) drinking two or three glasses of water (b) making a phone call to someone you love or makes you laugh (c) going for a brisk walk, or doing a work-out.

5. During your diet, it is advisable to practise the exercises in Chapter Eight, or to go swimming several times a week. You are the kind of person who enjoys sensual pleasures so have the occasional massage or sauna, and go to bed with a good, erotic book plus chocs from your allowance.

WEEK ONE

EVERY DAY Eat *one* Breakfast, *one* Light Meal, *one* Main Meal and *one* Treat.

BREAKFASTS (200 calories)
- 1 slice wholemeal toast, 1 size 3 poached egg, grilled tomato, watercress
- 1 large banana chopped up on top of 1oz (25g) unsweetened cereal, with milk from allowance
- 1 rasher well-grilled streaky bacon, 2oz (50g) sweetcorn, 2 crispbreads with a little low-fat spread, 1 small glass unsweetened apple or orange juice
- fruit salad of ½ medium melon, 1 small chopped banana, 2 fresh apricots, 2 tbsp yogurt, 1 tbsp mixed nuts

LUNCHES (300 calories)
Meals on Toast Top 2 slices wholemeal toast with one of the following:
- Lots of grilled tomatoes sprinkled with 1oz (25g) Edam cheese
- 1 small (5oz/125g) can baked beans, tomatoes, watercress
- ½ large can Heinz Weight Watchers Spaghetti
- 4oz (100g) mushrooms poached in chicken stock, 1 carton Shape or Diet Ski yogurt to follow

Salads Eat unlimited salad vegetables from your 'free' list (page 47) and choose one of the following accompaniments:
- 8oz (200g) chicken leg, no skin, 6oz (150g) jacket potato
- 2oz (50g) drained sardines, lemon juice, 1 Diet Ski or Shape yogurt, 1 small roll

- 2oz (50g) lean ham or smoked salmon (for a treat!), 1 slice wholemeal bread with low-fat spread, 1 large banana

Sandwiches 2 slices wholemeal bread, salad from 'free' list (page 47) and one of these fillings:

- 3oz (75g) tuna-in-brine
- 1 sliced hard-boiled egg
- 2oz (50g) cottage cheese with chopped gherkins and an apple to follow

SUPPERS (350 calories)
- 1 large slice melon, 10oz (250g) grilled trout or herring, huge salad from 'free' list, 1 small wholemeal roll
- ½ grapefruit with artificial sweetener, 3oz (75g) lean lamb chop, thin gravy, huge pile of vegetables from 'free' list, 1 scoop vanilla icecream with 4oz (100g) strawberries or raspberries
- Any Findus Lean Cuisine or Heinz Weight Watchers meal with huge pile of 'free' vegetables and salad
- Slimmer's soup, any flavour, any Bird's Eye fish in sauce meal, with vegetables and salad from 'free' list, 1 small banana, apple or pear
- Mixed grill of well-grilled beefburger, 4oz (100g) mushrooms cooked in chicken stock, grilled tomatoes, watercress, 1 grilled low-fat sausage, 3 tbsp baked beans. Add a huge mixed salad from 'free' list
- *Starter* of sliced tomatoes, 1oz (25g) cubed Edam cheese, chopped chives, with dressing of chopped garlic, vinegar and herbs; *main course* of 4oz (100g) chicken breast cooked in tin of low-calorie chicken soup, with vegetables from 'free' list; *dessert* of baked apple with a squirt of aerosol cream. Yum!
- 3oz (75g) any roast meat, thin gravy, 3oz (75g) chunks roast potato, huge helping of 'free' vegetables, red fruit

salad (1 sliced red apple, a few redcurrants, raspberries and strawberries) with 1 tbsp natural yogurt

TREATS   (100 calories) Choose *one* each day.
- 1 glass dry wine
- 2 pub-measure 'short' drinks with low-calorie mixers
- ½ pint beer or lager
- 1 large banana
- 1 digestive biscuit

WEEK TWO and subsequent weeks
Add your 300-calorie chocolate allowance just *three* times each day. Enjoy it without feeling guilty. Make sure you nibble each mouthful slowly. Alternatively include the recipes on page 117 onwards in your chocolate allowance, making sure you do not exceed your daily 300-calorie total.

DIET FOR WEEKEND INDULGERS
This diet allows 1000 calories on weekdays and 1400 calories on Saturdays and Sundays.

DAILY ALLOWANCES   ½ pint (275ml) skimmed milk for your tea and coffee, unlimited water and mineral water.

FREE VEGETABLES   You can eat as much as you like from the 'free' vegetable list page 47). You can boil or steam vegetables, or eat them raw. Do not use butter or margarine, and make your own dressing using lemon juice, vinegar, herbs and garlic.

- There is an alcohol allowance for weekends only.
- Do not add salt to cooking or sprinkle it on food.

STRATEGY
1. Make a list of the places where you normally buy

chocolate – the supermarket, garage or paper shop. Now, relax and imagine yourself going into each of these places without buying chocolate. Do this exercise every single day.

2.   Always carry fresh fruit in your car or bag, and eat it before going into a shop or during moments of tension.

3.   When you have chocs in the house, make sure they are kept out of sight in a tin on top of a cupboard.

4.   One of your problems is that you associate pleasure and treats with eating chocolates. So, every day give yourself a treat that doesn't involve eating, such as listening to music, reading a book, having a manicure or hair-do.

5.   When you go to a film or concert, make sure you eat a good meal before the show. Don't take chocs with you. Sit tight in the interval!

6.   You are a sensual person, so indulge in an occasional massage, using scented oils. It is fun to try this with a partner, especially if going to a salon seems too expensive.

7.   Get out into the fresh air at weekends. Take up a sport like golf, tennis, or just walk. Contrary to what most people think, exercise helps stop that choccy craving. Aim for 20 minutes of aerobic (swimming, cycling, exercise class) exercise every week.

WEEKDAYS
Choose *one* Breakfast, *one* Light Meal, *one* Main Meal and *one* Treat. Between meals, nibble anything you like from the 'free' vegetable list (page 47).

BREAKFASTS   (200 calories)
- 1oz (25g) any unsweetened cereal, milk from allowance, 1 large banana
- 1 size 3 egg, boiled or poached, 1 slice wholemeal toast with a little low-fat spread
- 1 slice melon, 1 slice wholemeal toast topped with 3oz

(75g) mushrooms, poached in chicken stock sprinkled with ½oz (12g) grated Edam cheese
- 1 Weetabix, milk from allowance, a few grapes, small glass orange juice

LIGHT MEALS   (250 calories)

Salads   Make a huge salad with vegetables from the 'free' list (page 47) and serve with one of these choices:
- 8oz (200g) chicken leg, no skin, grilled or roast, 1 apple or orange
- 4oz (100g) steamed or grilled fish, 1 small boiled potato, 1 small banana
- 1 small carton cottage cheese, 2 tbsp sweetcorn, 2 chopped apricots, 1 slice wholemeal bread

Sandwiches   2 two slices wholemeal bread with salad from 'free' list (page 47) and one of these fillings:
- 1 small, chopped banana with lemon juice
- 1 tsp peanut butter
- 1 cold, chopped chipolata sausage
- 1 chopped apple with ½oz (12g) mixed nuts

Soups
- 1 tin slimmer's soup, any flavour, 1 slice wholemeal bread, 1 carton Diet Ski or Shape Yogurt
- Home-made vegetable soup (use vegetables from 'free' list) with wholemeal croutons, 1 slice toast topped with tomatoes, a few grapes

MAIN MEALS   (400 calories)

Don't forget to pile on the 'free' salads and vegetables.
- Any Findus Lean Cuisine or Heinz Weight Watchers Meal with 1 apple, orange or small banana to follow
- 3oz (75g) (cooked weight) wholemeal pasta or wholegrain rice with one of the following toppings plus 1 small wholemeal roll and an apple or orange to follow:

- 3oz (75g) prawns with tomatoes, herbs, garlic
- 1oz (25g) chopped ham with tin of slimmer's mushroom soup
- 4oz (100g) liver, grilled with thin gravy, 1 rasher streaky bacon, grilled, 1 beef chipolata sausage, grilled, 3oz (75g) mashed potato, 4oz (100g) mushrooms poached in water, grilled tomatoes
- 8oz (200g) chicken leg, no skin, 3oz (75g) (cooked weight) wholegrain rice, 2oz (50g) sweetcorn, 2oz (50g) carrots
- 3oz (75g) any lean roast meat, thin gravy, 2 medium chunks roast potato, 2oz (50g) peas, 1oz (25g) scoop vanilla icecream
- 1 can slimmer's soup, any flavour, 4oz (100g) trout or herring, grilled, 2 small boiled potatoes, 2oz (50g) carrots, 1 carton Diet Ski or Shape yogurt

TREATS   (50 calories) Choose *one* each day.
- 1 small digestive biscuit
- 2 crispbreads with a little low-fat spread and sliced tomatoes
- 1 small banana

WEEKENDS
As for weekdays, but, after the first week, add 300 calories worth of chocolates *daily* from the list on page 140, **OR** 300 calories worth of recipes from Chapter Ten.
You may also have one of the following each day:
- 1 glass dry wine
- 2 pub-measure 'short' drinks with low-calorie mixers
- ½ pint beer or lager

EATING OUT
Choose clear soup or melon, then a simple fish or meat dish, with vegetables and salads. At Indian restaurants go for

chicken tikka or tandoori, cucumber riata, poppadam and plain boiled rice. At Italian restaurants choose fish, cooked simply without sauces. Carvery choices should be turkey with fresh vegetables and a small icecream to follow.

DIET FOR SUGAR ADDICTS

Please note: it is very likely that you will need additional counselling and help with your slimming campaign. Do have a check up with your doctor and also consult the list of eating disorders counselling services on page 154. If in doubt, do write to me at the address on page 154.

DAILY ALLOWANCES ½ pint (275ml) skimmed milk for your tea and coffee, unlimited water and mineral water. Try to limit cups of tea and coffee to two a day, and try to drink herb tea instead. Drink lots of water.

FREE VEGETABLES Eat as much as you like from the 'free' vegetable list (page 47). Boil or steam vegetables, or serve them raw as salads. Do not add butter or oil. Instead, make your own dressing with lemon juice, vinegar, herbs and garlic.

CHOCOLATE After the first week, you may have 200 calories of chocolate every day (*see* list on page 140 or the recipes in Chapter Ten). Eat it slowly and enjoy it.

• Do not add salt in cooking or sprinkle it on food.

STRATEGY

1. Take up yoga or meditation to help you cope. There are a number of good classes to go to – enquire locally.
2. Walk briskly for 20 minutes each day to help beat stress and rev up your metabolism. Even if you are in the kind of job where you use up a lot of energy rushing around, it is still

important to walk. You may think you are 'on the go' all day long, but you are in fact getting little *real* exercise.

3. Make sure you eat regularly. The diet gives you four meals a day, plus treats. Spread them out, so your blood sugar level is kept high. Missing meals is dangerous, both for your health and your slimming campaign.

4. Keep fresh fruit with you at all times to nibble when you feel low or tired.

5. Take a multi-vitamin capsule every day. Before a period, women can include Vitamin B6 and Evening Primrose oil capsules.

6. When you have time off work get plenty of fresh air – walk, play tennis, swim.

7. Make a list of all the places you usually buy chocolates, and avoid them. Buy your chocolate allowance from somewhere different and get it every day, not in huge quantities.

WEEK ONE

EVERYDAY Eat *one* Breakfast, *two* Light Meals, *one* Main Meal and *one* Treat every day.

BREAKFASTS (150 calories)
- 1 huge slice melon, 1 slice wholemeal toast topped with 2 tbsp cottage cheese
- 1oz (25g) any unsweetened cereal, milk from allowance, 1 small banana
- 1 carton natural yogurt with chopped apple and a sprinkling of nuts
- 2 crispbreads topped with 2 tsps peanut butter and sliced tomatoes
- 1 sandwich of 2 slices slimmer's bread, tomatoes, ½oz (12g) grated Edam cheese

LIGHT MEALS   (200 calories each)

Jacket potatoes   Cook a 5oz (125g) jacket potato and serve with salad and one of the following:

- 1oz (25g) chopped ham or chicken
- 2 tbsp baked beans
- 1 carton Shape coleslaw

Meals on toast   Top 1 slice wholemeal toast with one of the following, and add a large mixed salad:

- 2oz (50g) sardines, drained of oil
- 1 small (5oz/125g) tin baked beans
- 1 grilled fish cake
- 1 size 3 egg, poached

Salads   Make a huge mixed salad from the 'free' vegetable list (page 47) and add one of these accompaniments:

- 2oz (50g) cold chicken (no skin), 2 tbsp sweetcorn, 1 apple or orange
- 1 sliced size 3 egg, 1 crusty wholemeal roll
- 4oz (100g) grilled fish, 1 slice wholemeal bread
- 2oz (50g) corned beef, 1 medium banana

Sandwiches   2 slices wholemeal bread, salad from the 'free' list (page 47) and one of the following:

- 2 tbsp cottage cheese
- 1 small chopped banana
- 2oz (50g) tuna-in-brine

MAIN MEALS   (350 calories)

Add plenty of 'free' vegetables (page 47) and salads.

- Any Findus Lean Cuisine or Heinz Weight Watchers Meal
- 5oz (125g) lean lamb chop, 17½oz (215g) can wholewheat spaghetti topped with sliced tomato, 1oz (25g) grated Shape cheddar cheese, small bunch grapes
- 1 large slice of melon, 3oz (25g) canned sardines on 1 slice toast, grilled tomatoes, watercress, 1 orange
- 5oz (125g) grilled herring or tinned pilchards, 2 small

boiled potatoes, 1 serving Bird's Lite Mousse
- 1 well-grilled beefburger, 2 tbsp sweetcorn, 5oz (125g) jacket potato, 4oz (100g) strawberries or raspberries
- 4oz (100g) grilled liver, thin gravy, with 2 tbsp fresh orange juice added, 2 small boiled potatoes, 2 tbsp sweetcorn or peas, 1 apple
- 8oz (200g) chicken leg, no skin, grilled or roast with 5oz (125g) jacket potato topped with 1 tbsp cottage cheese
- 6oz (150g) any grilled white fish, 3oz (75g) potatoes mashed with skimmed milk from allowance, 2 tbsp sweetcorn or carrots, 1 apple or orange

TREATS (100 calories) Choose *one* each day.
- ½ pint beer or lager
- 1 glass dry wine
- 2 pub-measure 'short' drinks with low-calorie mixers
- 1 large digestive biscuit
- 2 crispbreads topped with cottage cheese and sliced tomato
- 1 large banana

WEEK TWO and subsequent weeks
Add 200 calories of chocolate (*see* list on page 140), **OR** *200 calories of desserts or drinks from the recipes on pages 117-135.*

CHAPTER SEVEN

OUR SUCCESS STORIES

The Chocoholic Diet was tested on groups of real-life chocolate addicts. Our volunteers were brave enough to be weighed, questioned and photographed over a period of four months. It is thanks to them that my team was able to try out the six versions of the diet and make any necessary changes to the eating programme.

We asked each volunteer to keep a weekly diary of their food intake, choccy cravings, and mood swings which we examined at every meeting. It is a good idea for all slimmers to do this, as it does help to pinpoint particular times of day when you are most vulnerable. It also helps you to understand why you turn to chocolate at difficult moments. Our volunteers were able to discuss their diaries with myself and Jan Long who is one of my top slimming counsellors.

If you keep a similar diary, read it through each week quietly when you are alone, or alternatively ask a sympathetic friend to go through it with you. Check the do-it-yourself diary analysis chart on page 137, and you will be able to identify problems and, hopefully, solve them!

Most of our volunteers had 'hiccups' right at the very beginning of their slimming campaign. When you have been dependent on an emotional and physical prop which is as powerful as chocolate, controlling your dependency is obviously going to be difficult. But, in every case, the choccy cravings did go away and the volunteers did lose weight. The six volunteers below are now able to eat chocolate in moderation without bingeing.

In each case there was a turning point where the slimmer suddenly found that he or she felt stronger and more in control of their bodies and minds. This was very much associated with the benefits of the good nutrition they had been enjoying on the diet; once you feel stronger and can see the benefits of good, regular meals, you will be well on the way to permanent weight-loss.

One point to note is that our slimmers had problems when they ate less than the amount of food and drink specified in the diet. It is very important indeed to eat enough – if you don't you, too, will come unstuck. Eating too little is counter-productive: you may certainly lose weight more quickly, but you will be unable to carry on with the diet for very long, and will almost certainly binge. Even if this doesn't happen, cutting calories too low will make your body go into 'starvation mode', and when you do start eating again you will get even fatter than you were before. Honestly!

Name: **Wendi Cook**
Age: 25   *Height*: 5ft 4in
Occupation: Full-time mother   *From*: Strood, Kent
Starting weight: **14st 6lb**   *Weight after 20 Weeks*: **13st**
Weight after 28 weeks: **12st 7lb**   *Diet Plan*: Comfort Eater

Pretty Wendi has two children aged 6 and 4. Her husband often works away from home. Her chocolate addiction started as a 'comfort', filling the lonely gaps when she was on her own. 'I was eating around six bars of solid chocolate daily – such as Galaxy – supplementing it with other foods containing chocolate. Things like Bandits which are chocolate-covered wafer biscuits were always in my kitchen.'

Wendi stashed away her chocolate supplies in an unusual place – her childrens' toy cupboard. 'I would pop smaller, funsize Mars and Snickers bars in there among the dolls and toy cars. When the children went to the cupboard, I'd sit down and watch them play, eating the chocolates at the same time.'

'If we went out shopping, I would always want some kind of chocolate snack, such as a knickerbocker glory, or a chocolate doughnut. It was absolutely ridiculous to be spending so much money on chocolate, and it was doing awful things to my figure, so I realised that I would have to kick the habit.'

When Wendi came to our group, she felt tired and low. 'I was fed up with wearing baggy clothes and being out of breath. I knew I had to lose at least a stone or so, but didn't see how I could beat my chocolate addiction.'

The first week was encouraging, and Wendi lost 3lb. Here is her diary for the first few days of the week:

MONDAY
Breakfast 1oz cereal, milk, apple, 2 crispbreads with a little low-fat spread. Comments: 'This is a lot more than I normally eat, and it's hard to find time to eat it with the children to sort out. But I felt very full afterwards and didn't want any chocolate.'

Light Meal Ham sandwich with large portion of salad. Comments: 'I'm not wild about salad, but this tasted fresh and I enjoyed the sandwich.'

Main Meal Grilled liver, mushrooms, green beans, jacket potato. Comments: 'This was very satisfying. I was with the children, and they enjoyed it too.'

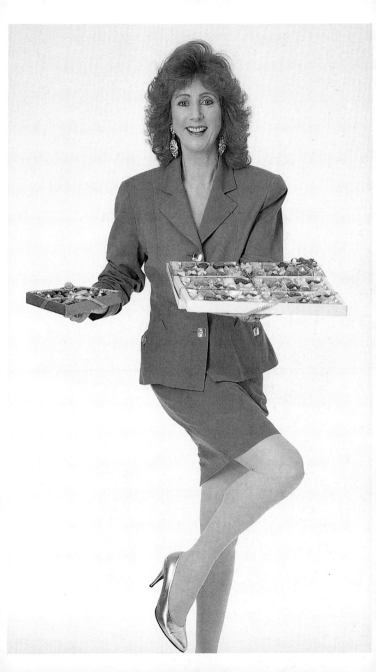

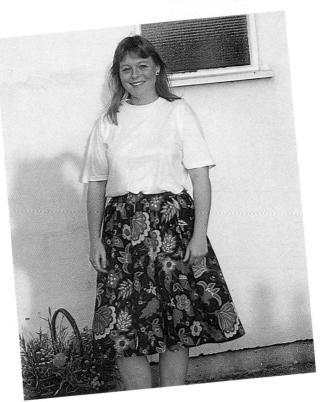

Before

Community midwife Janice Spencer, 32, was a chocoholic teenager and her nursing career made her problems even worse :

"It's so easy to scoff chocs on night-duty," she says. "Patients give them to the staff, and they are left around for everyone to nibble. As a chocoholic, I was faced with temptation every single day."

Now glamorous Janice, who has two young children as well as a busy working life, has shrunk from 10st 8lb to 9st 5lb - perfect for her height of five feet two inches".

She says : "I am determined to stay in shape - the diet is so easy to stick to, and I feel just great."

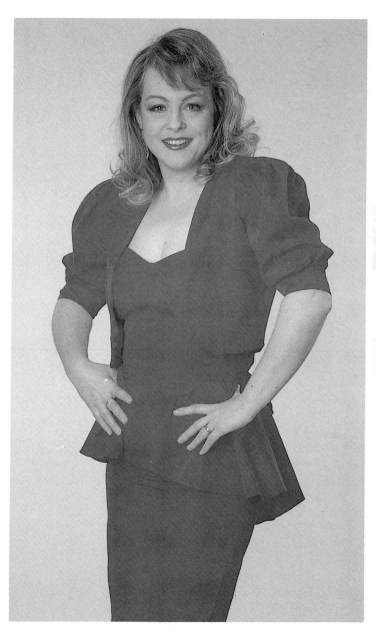

After

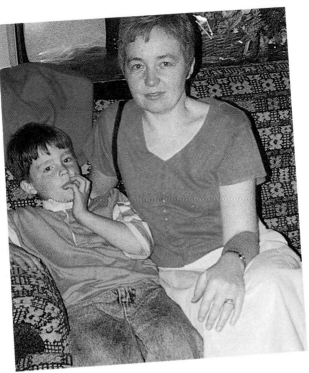

Before

It's hard to imagine that pretty Josie Kirby, 39, is the mother of two teenagers.

She's a slim, trim 9st 4lbs - perfect for her height of five feet four inches.

Yet, before she started on *The Chocoholic Diet*, she was tired, run-down and weighed in at 10st 8lb.

She says : I ate chocolate in secret, to help me cope with pressure. Now, I can eat it openly and enjoy every mouthful without binging."

Josie finds that she can pack far more into her life these days. "I go to aerobics classes, which have helped tone up my body. They also give me lots of energy," she says.

She is now following *The Chocoholic Diet* maintenance plan, to keep her weight steady. "I feel terrific, and much more in control, these days."

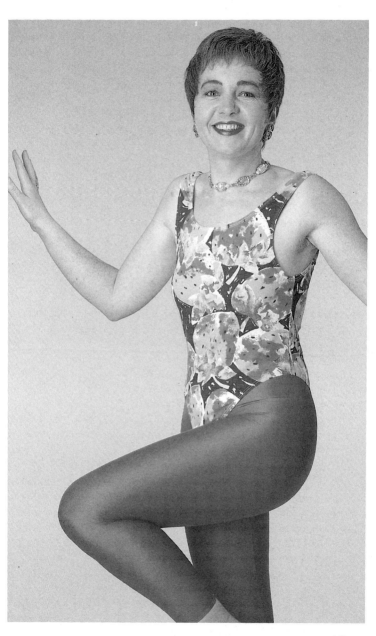

After

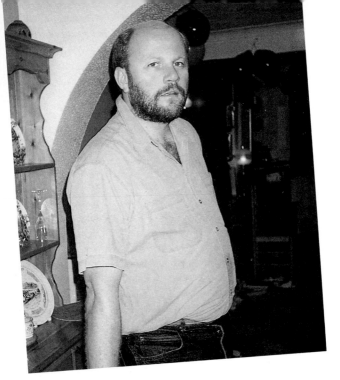

Before

Businessman David Herron, 38, was a five feet ten and a half inch tall, 16st 3lb sitting target for the fat-traps which lie in wait for male chocoholics.

He works long hours in a highly demanding job, and there is a constant supply of junk food and confectionery in and around his office.

"Most of my chocoholic attacks happened at work," he says. "There's a vending machine near my office. I was drawn to it like a magnet."

When he switched to *The Chocoholic Diet*, he actually ate *more* than ever before, and craved fewer chocs. He also worked off his problems - and his waistline - by pedalling away furiously on a cycling machine in front of the TV.

In just a few months, David lost two stone, and now tips the scales at 14st 3lb

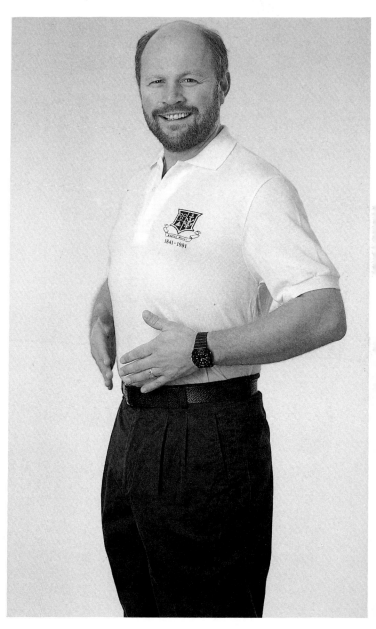

After

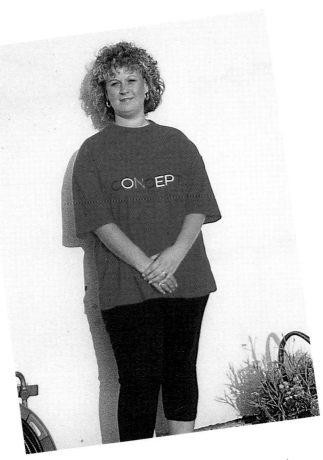

Before

Curvy Christine Ryan, 25, has a year old baby and looks a million dollars. But when she started *The Chocoholic Diet*, she weighed in at 13st, and was furious with herself for putting on 4 and a half stone during her pregnancy.

"I didn't realise that it would be so hard to shed the extra weight after my baby was born," she says. "I seemed to crave more and more chocolate, night and day." Now, Christine is down to 11 and a half stone and still losing. She is determined to shed at least another stone.

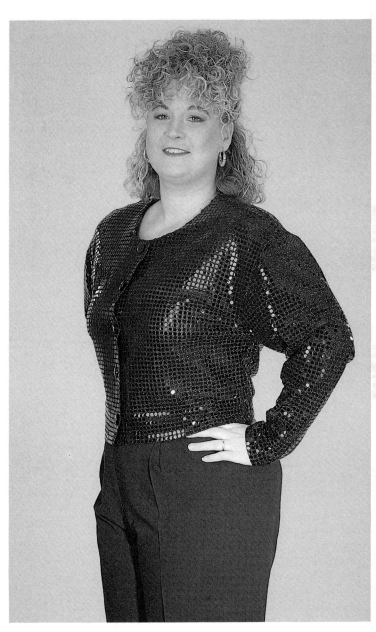

After

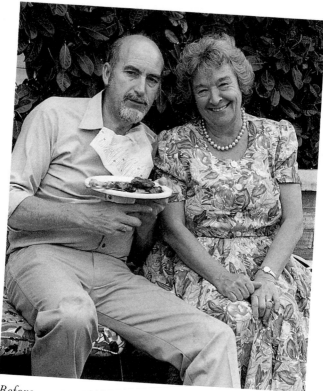

Before

Bubbly Betty Gower, 62, is a glamorous granny who stocked up with chocs to give her grandchildren - then ate them herself.

"It took this picture of me with a friend, looking huge in that flowered dress, to make me realise that 13 st 3 lb was too heavy for my five feet four inch frame," says Betty. She was given extra weekend rations of chocolate on her version of *The Chocoholic Diet*, and now she has lost more than a stone.

"I couldn't believe how much better I would feel with just a 16 lb weight loss," she says. "I am now determined to shed another stone. It's nice to know that I'll be able to eat chocolate while I carry on slimming."

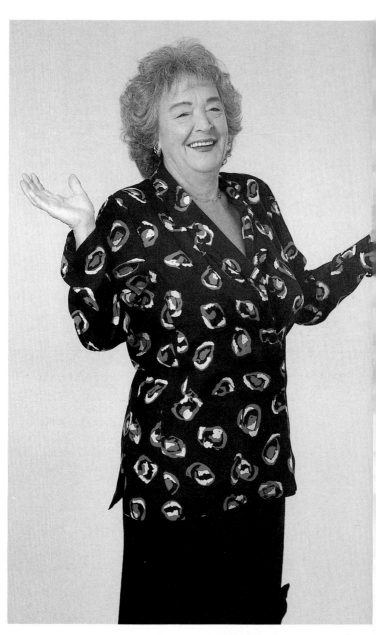

After

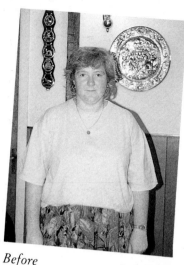

Before

Pretty Wendi Cook, 25, was bored with being a dumpy 14st 6lb.

"I couldn't wear trendy clothes and hide my bulges under baggy skirts and oversized T-shirts," she says.

Now she weighs 12 and a half stone and is shedding weight at the rate of around 2lbs weekly.

Her 'goal' is 10st." I used to hide bars of chocolate among my children's toys and sneak a few bites at playtime," she says.

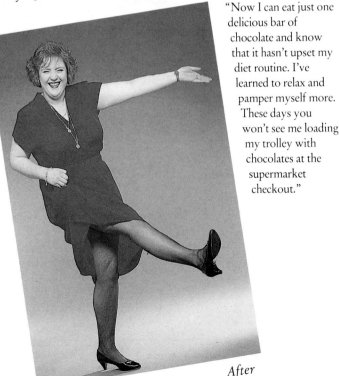

"Now I can eat just one delicious bar of chocolate and know that it hasn't upset my diet routine. I've learned to relax and pamper myself more. These days you won't see me loading my trolley with chocolates at the supermarket checkout."

After

Treats 1 banana, crispbreads with cottage cheese. Comments: 'Today, it was a real challenge not to go to my usual shops for chocolate. I quite enjoyed the feeling of control. But how long will it last? Predictably, the hardest bit was in the evening so I had my snacks then. Why do they have so many chocolate commercials on TV?'

TUESDAY
Breakfast 1 egg, slice of toast. Comments: 'I was tempted to forget the egg, but made time for it. Will I ever get used to these breakfasts?'

Lunch Chicken sandwich, with salad. Comments: 'I'm getting bored with the lunch, will have something different tomorrow. It's fun stopping myself from going out for chocolates. I did some exercises instead!'

Supper Pasta with prawns and tomatoes, 1 apple. 'I want more – but still have my snacks left, so that's okay. On the whole, I feel I am doing well. Let's see what the scales say at the end of the week. I definitely won't be tempted to weigh myself until then.'

Treats Nimble bread with salad, 1 banana. Comments: 'Had a glass of Martini as well, but stopped at that. This is going well'.

Wendi could probably have lost a little more weight the first week, but she cut back on breakfast against our instructions, and found herself eating sauté potatoes in the evening! However, the second week she was able to introduce chocolate without bingeing:

'I started with Jaffa Cakes, which are only 45 calories each, so I could have four every day,' she says. 'I felt it was still too early to tempt fate by buying chocolate bars. Following your advice, I would save the Jaffa Cakes for times during the day when I could really enjoy them. I would make myself a cup of tea or coffee, and take it into the sitting room, with one Jaffa Cake only, then sit down and eat it slowly, savouring the runny orange bit in the middle. Before, I would do most of my choc-nibbling in the kitchen and gobble a whole packet of chocolate biscuits at one go!'

Here is an example from one of Wendi's more recent diaries:

SATURDAY:

Breakfast Toast, tomatoes, cheese. 'I feel really great, and don't want chocolate. I want to make it to 13 stone 7lb on my next weigh-in and I think I can do it.'

Lunch Jacket potato with baked beans, and a huge salad. 'We all went shopping, but I took some fruit with me. I bought Caramac bars for the children, but did not want to buy one for myself. I bought a new blouse instead.'

Supper Quiche, salad, another jacket potato. 'I am adapting the diet to suit myself, but I must watch quiches – as they can be higher in calories than you imagine. I had 200 calories worth of chocolate stored in the tin I use for this. It was there if I wanted it – but I only ate one fun-size Mars, then put it back. I really didn't want the rest.'

Treats Spritzer (white wine and soda water), crispbreads with cottage cheese. 'I finally ate my Mars bar very slowly while I was drinking the spritzer and watching TV. It tasted very wicked and luxurious!'

SUNDAY:

Breakfast Cereal, milk, apple, crispbreads. 'Sunday is

normally very bad for me, so I have lined up lots of jobs to do today.'

Lunch Chicken casserole, lots of vegetables, mashed potato. 'I still have chocolate left from yesterday's allowance, but would rather have some fruit after lunch. I am winning!'

Supper Large salad, cottage cheese, sweetcorn. 'Now, I do fancy the chocs, but I will save them for later on. Maybe I'll have a chocolate drink in bed. Tried on the blouse I bought yesterday. It looked great!'

As you can see from our photographs, Wendy is now looking super. She is still following the diet, and intends to hit her 'goal' weight of 10st 10lb by the summer, when she will go on our maintenance plan.

'The most difficult thing was to convince my husband that I can now have chocolate. He generally teases me if he sees me eating it. But, I think he'll get the message soon!'

Name: **Josie Kirby**
Age: 36   *Height*: 5ft 6in
Occupation: Office Worker   *From*: South East London
Starting weight: **10st 8lb**   *Weight after 20 weeks*: **9st 8lb**
Weight after 28 weeks: **9st 4lb** *Diet Plan*: Secret Binger

Josie was very tired and run down when she joined our chocoholics group in Bexleyheath, Kent. She is a hard-working mum, with two teenage children. Divorced, she now lives with her boyfriend and they are getting married later this year.

Josie admits that she ate chocolate in secret because she found it hard to cope with the pressures of life. 'I am probably typical of many women trying to do their best for everyone. We should realise that it just isn't possible!'

She would buy chocolate on the way to or from work, put it in her shopping bag, and eat it at home in the bathroom or her bedroom. 'My binges usually coincided with tension at home. Every teenager in the world is untidy but when you come back exhausted after a busy day at work, something snaps when you find the flat in a mess. I'm no different from any mum but I just dealt with the problem the wrong way. I was punishing myself, instead of discussing things rationally with the family.'

We advised Josie to give herself more treats. In particular, we suggested that she started going to a weekly fitness class since exercise is a great outlet for stress and helps reduce carbohydrate cravings. We also had a good chat (and a few moans!) about the problems of coping with family pressures, which did Josie a lot of good. Remember, like her, you are not alone. (Do write to me at the address on page 154 if you feel you want to get something off your chest and can't find anyone else to listen. It is better to bitch than binge!)

Josie started her diet feeling very positive. Here is an extract from one of her early diaries:

FRIDAY:
Breakfast Cereal, milk, chopped banana. Comment: 'I made time to pack up some fruit and a cottage cheese sandwich for lunch. Felt fine.'

Lunch Cottage cheese sandwich, salad. Comment: 'Ate this after my aerobics class. We did stepping exercises today which were fun. But during the afternoon, I suddenly found myself fantasying about all the chocolate bars I used to eat – from Fruit and Nut to Mars. Had a piece of fruit, quickly.'

Early evening Slimmer's soup, wholemeal bread, carton of yogurt. Comment: 'I suddenly realised that I had no chocolates to eat, so went to the kitchen to make this snack, which I am allowed on my diet. It was very satisfying!'

Supper Melon, sardines on toast, salad, grilled tomatoes, 1 orange. Comment: 'So far, so good. Everything is fine, and I don't feel irritable or tired.'

Treats Crispbread with cottage cheese, and another mug of soup at bedtime. Comment: 'If I can do this, I will be surprised. That fantasy list of chocs kept on bugging me all evening. I could see them waiting for me at my local sweetshop!'

SATURDAY

Breakfast Cereal, with milk. Comment: 'No time for anything else, I am going shopping and then on to help with my sister's children's birthday party at a local swimming pool.'

Lunch Salad sandwich. Comment: 'In a hurry, should have eaten more. I forgot to bring anything suitable to eat with me and felt weak with hunger during the afternoon. I had a slice of birthday cake and found I didn't enjoy it as much as I thought I would.'

Supper Egg roll, another cottage cheese and salad sandwich and 4 vodkas. Comment: 'Help! I hope I'm not going to turn into an alcoholic instead of a chocoholic. I will try harder to eat correctly tomorrow.'

Josie made the classic mistake of missing out on food, just when she needed it most – on the day she was helping with the children's pool party. But, this experience taught her to be prepared. Here's an extract from one of her later diaries:

MONDAY

Breakfast Cereal, chopped apple, milk. Comment: 'This week, I am determined to do well. I feel much better since going regularly to my aerobics class. My mother baked two cakes at the weekend, a fruit cake and a chocolate log. I picked at both of them, but didn't wolf down the chocolate one as I would have done before starting the diet.'

Lunch Tuna and salad sandwich, banana. 'I will make sure I don't leave too long a gap between meals, and go for a walk tonight.'

Early Evening 1 slice toast topped with tomatoes and grated Edam cheese. 'I nibbled this snack while preparing the family's supper. Delicious.'

Supper 5oz lamb chop, thin gravy, 3oz mashed potato made with milk from allowance, a glass of dry wine. Comment: 'It seems as though I've eaten a lot today. I could have 150 calories worth of chocolate tonight, but am not sure I need it ... will decide later. Tried on size 12 jeans. They fit – hurrah!'

TUESDAY

Breakfast Cereal, banana. Comment: 'Still thrilled about the jeans. My thighs look so much slimmer. Everyone's commenting.'

Lunch Cottage cheese roll, fruit. Comment: 'I enjoy taking my lunch into the park. It's good to get away from pressures in the fresh air.'

Early Evening Home-made vegetable soup, wholemeal croutons. Comment: 'Tried on some knickers, size 38-40, bought today – they were too big. Things are definitely looking good.'

Supper Findus Lean Cuisine meal, huge pile of 'free' vegetables, 1 banana. 'Family atmosphere is good, and I'm looking forward to a trip to Ireland. Wonder how I will cope with all the food?'

In fact, Josie coped extremely well on her holiday. 'My taste-buds seem to be tuned-in to fresher foods, fruits, salads and vegetables, so I really wasn't turned on by the heavier Irish dishes. To my amazement, I didn't gain weight at all, even though we celebrated Christmas in the middle of my holiday – with all the chocolate temptations around.'

Josie's most difficult time was when she was called for Jury Service. 'All chocoholics should be warned that sheer frustration can set you craving chocs while you are spending long hours waiting to go into court. There is so much hanging about that the whole thing drives you nuts. You want to do your duty, but you have to fall in with a system which is not designed for impatient people.'

'It is also very stressful, because the cases are often harrowing.'

Josie coped by taking food with her, plus plenty to read and a portable radio with a Walkman so she could tune in when waiting between court appearances.

She has now reached her 'goal' weight, and looks terrific. She is convinced that her bingeing days are well and truly over!

Name: **David Herron**
Age: 38   *Height*: 5ft 10½in

Occupation: Manager, air express company
From: Welling, Kent
Starting weight: **16st 3lb**   *Weight after 10 weeks*: **14st 10lb**
Weight after 25 weeks: **14st 3lb**   *Diet Plan*: Comfort Eater

Dave Herron is married with one child. His wife works as a midwife and is a wonderful cook! However, Dave's chocoholism was triggered more by the nature and location of his work than the food he eats at home.

He says, 'My office is very handy for comfort eating – it's near a whole load of fast-food places, confectionery shops and restaurants. There's even a chocolate vending machine on the wall near my office.'

Dave has to deal with clients all day long, some of them difficult, so it was all too easy to get a quick 'fix' of chocolate when things got tough. When he came along to our chocoholic group, he was consuming around 4500 calories a day and a great deal of that was in the form of chocolate. His favourites? Mars, Fruit & Nut, chocolate chip cookies, and his wife's amazing chocolate cake.

Here is a typical day's food and drink for Dave, before he started the Chocoholic Diet:

Breakfast   Cereal or 3 or 4 slices of toast and marmalade

Snack   (sometimes on the way to work) Bar of chocolate, doughnut

Lunch   2 or 3 rolls with butter and meat filling, chocolate bar

Mid-Afternoon   2 or 3 chocolate bars

After work   2 or 3 pints of lager and a burger

Supper   Large cooked dinner, followed by a pudding, and more chocolate

82

Not surprisingly, Dave was gaining weight fast. He says, 'I looked in the mirror one day and decided that enough was enough. But I was worried about just how I was going to beat the fast-food trap and control my chocolate cravings.'

We advised Dave to eat a substantial breakfast and bring a packed lunch to work, at least until he began to control his eating pattern. He threw himself into the plan with tremendous enthusiasm, peddling away on a cycling machine in front of the TV every night to burn off extra calories.

The first week, he lost a massive 8lb! Then his weight stayed the same for one week. 'I found this very annoying, until I remembered that I had had a very stupid day on the Sunday. My wife had been at the hospital all day, and I had been cooking for myself and my daughter. Frankly, I had pigged-out between meals – perhaps because I was feeling a bit sorry for myself. I had tried so hard to curb my choc-oholism during the week, that I let myself go on that particular day.'

Gradually, Dave learned to monitor his own food intake and to allow himself the occasional chocolate treat as well as some fast food. He can now work out, roughly, the calorie count of his daily meals, snacks and drinks, and makes sure that over a few days it balances out at roughly 1750-2000 calories, which is about right for him.

He deals with problems as they arise and pedals away the stresses of the day on his exercise bike. He feels younger, fitter and swears that he will never go back to his former eating habits.

Here is a typical two-day food diary from his new regime, with his comments:

FRIDAY
Breakfast   3 Weetabix, semi-skimmed milk, coffee.

10.30 am   Lo Fruit Bar   *11.30 am*   Lo Choc Bar

Comments: 'I now always eat a very substantial breakfast, with plenty of fibre. If I have time, I will have something cooked, but I find that 3 Weetabix – which don't have sugar added – is a satisfying start to the day. Lo Bars are good because they contain just over 100 calories, so I can have two for my daily choc allowance.'

Lunch   1 crusty roll with cold low-fat pork sausage and salad filling, plus a large extra portion of mixed salad with lots of raw vegetables in a bowl with a little low-calorie mayonnaise. Comments: 'I find that this lunch fills me up more than a fast food item like a pie or burger,' he says. 'I no longer get hunger pains in the afternoons.'

After work   2½ pints of lager. 'I now look on my beer as a food, not just a drink. I didn't realise that the calories it contains put weight on. I just thought it was liquid retention that caused a beer belly!'

Supper   1 medium Deep Pan Pizza with Pepperoni and Ham. 'This is a high-calorie snack, but fairly moderate as a main meal for a man my size,' he says. 'These days, I wouldn't dream of having a pizza as well as a normal meal.'

SATURDAY

Brunch   1 wholemeal roll, with 1oz ham and Shape Low Fat Cheese Spread, tall glass of tomato juice. 'If you wake late on Saturday, it makes sense to have a late breakfast. I was full after last night's pizza!'

Teatime   Heinz Weight Watchers Soup, crispbread, Findus Lean Cuisine ready meal, large portion of vegetables from the 'free' list, 1 apple, Diet Lilt. 'This was very healthy and filling, and easy to prepare too. I felt like going for a walk afterwards, instead of collapsing into a chair!'

Evening   1½ cans of Stella lager

Late Night Snack   More soup, crusty roll, banana. 'I never even thought about chocolate today, so I have saved my allowance in a tin for tomorrow – but maybe I won't want it then, who knows?'

Dave's next big test will come when he goes on holiday or gets away from his routine. He has definitely sorted out his problems at work and at home. Luckily, he now looks so good in tight-fitting t-shirts that vanity should help to keep him on the straight and narrow. Check out his 'before and after' photographs.

Name: **Christine Ryan**
Age: 25   *Height*: 5ft 2in
Occupation: Customer Service Clerk   *From*: Welling, Kent
Starting weight: **13 stone**   *Weight after 20 weeks*: **12 stone**
Weight after 28 weeks: **11st 7lb**
Diet Plans: Premenstrual Craver and Comfort Eater

Christine had a one-year old baby when she started the Chocoholic Diet. She had begun her pregnancy weighing 10 stone and expanded to 14½ stone during the nine months. Afterwards, despite trying to diet, she had not managed to slim down below 13 stone and she was worried that she would never regain her pre-baby figure.

'My chocoholism was much worse when I was pregnant,' she says. 'I craved chocolate bars night and day. Unfortunately, I thought I'd be able to get away with eating so much so long as I went on a diet afterwards. I never revealed to the hospital gynaecologist this problem, and he didn't nag me to lose weight, so I thought I was fine. I was lucky not to suffer any complications.'

Christine breast-fed her baby for six weeks and managed to lose half a stone, but then found that her weight crept up again. Her worst chocolate orgies seemed to be associated with hormone activity – she ate more during the week before her monthly period.

'My husband is out usually three nights each week, and on those nights I would eat three or four bars of chocolate while watching television. I'd also keep a large pack of fun-size bars in the fridge, and eat one every time I went there to get food for the baby.'

She bought most of her chocs at her local supermarket, pretending to herself that they were for her slimline husband, 'I was sincerely trying to lose weight after having my son, but kidding myself every inch of the way,' she says. 'My husband is slim and in a high-energy job and adores chocs too. The problem is that he burns off all the calories and I don't. I would put the chocolate bars in the fridge, sincerely believing that the whole pack was for him and gradually eat my way through it!'

Christine's haywire hormones made her very aware of the problem so many chocoholics face – chocs are everywhere! 'Chemist shops display them right by the prescription counter, you have to walk past chocs before you buy your cinema ticket, you can't even take children to a swimming pool without running the gauntlet of vending machines displaying chocolate snacks. I used to try everything to avoid them but it was as though some unseen force was propelling me towards these displays.'

When she joined the chocoholic group, Christine was full of determination. We gave her two plans: the Five-Meal-a-Day

Premenstrual Cravers diet for the week of her monthly cycle which was particularly difficult, with the Comfort Eaters' diet for the rest of the month.

Christine's husband kindly offered to stop eating chocs in front of her, and encouraged her all the way. She started off very well indeed, losing an amazing 5lb in the first week. Here is the first day of her food diary:

MONDAY

Breakfast ½ grapefruit, cereal, banana, milk. 'I am determined to lose weight on this diet. Sounds like a typical Monday morning vow of determination. Will I stick to it?'

Snack 2 thin slices wholemeal bread with salad and cottage cheese. 'Nice and tasty – so far, so good!'

Lunch Large mixed salad, 3oz chicken, 2 tbsp sweetcorn, 1 apple. 'I seem to have been eating all day. I like this. No choc cravings yet.'

Snack 4oz figs, canned in syrup, sprinkled with 1 tbsp unsweetened muesli and topped with a carton of natural yogurt. 'A nice sweet-tasting treat.'

Supper Findus Lean Cuisine Cod Mornay, broccoli, green beans, grapes. 'Hard not to reach for a choc during the evening, maybe tomorrow I will have one of my snacks later. However, I can have a carton of fromage frais and a biscuit later on, so it's not too bad.'

After starting off so well, Christine suffered a 'hiccup' around the pre-Christmas period, when she was very busy. 'I put a few pounds back on mainly because I didn't have time to eat enough of the right food ... and found myself wanting chocolate,' she says.

She went back onto the diet in January with new determination. However, on inspection of her food diary, we found that she wasn't eating enough. Here is an extract:

MONDAY
Breakfast 2 slices toast. 'It's all I've got time for'.

Lunch Chicken, salad. 'Still feel hungry and fancy an Aero bar.'

Supper Salmon steak, large portion green vegetables, small potato.

Snack 1 glass wine. 'Didn't give into Aero craving... well done!'

Not surprisingly, by the end of the week, she *had* given into that Aero craving and had polished off 4 fingers of Kit Kat and a Cadbury's Flake as well! When she studied her diary, Christine realised that she was eating too little and not having enough for breakfast. Chocoholics need a protein food, such as an egg, cottage cheese or a yogurt, early in the day. She now makes sure that she eats regularly and well. Things are looking up, and at the last weigh-in, Christine had lost 21lb, and felt just great.

Name: **Janice Spencer**
Age: 32   *Height*: 5ft 2in
Occupation: Community Midwife   *From*: Welling, Kent
Starting weight: **10st 8lb**   *Weight after 20 Weeks*: **9st 11lb**
Weight after 28 weeks: **9st 4lb**   *Diet Plan*: Comfort Eater

Janice is a girl with a lot of responsibilities. She has two children aged 5 and 18 months, and is also a community midwife. She comes from a family who enjoy their chocs; her mother, Lynne, is a choc and sweet-eating champion!

'I started to put on weight as a teenager, and left school weighing around 10 stone,' she says. 'When I was a student nurse, it was very difficult to eat regular meals. We were all learning the principles of good nutrition, then eating chocolate bars to give us the energy to keep going.

'I got into the habit of eating chocolate on night duty. People give nurses boxes of sweets and chocolates all the time, so if you're a chocoholic life is very difficult indeed. The very first thing you see when you walk into the office is a box of unopened Black Magic or Milk Tray on the desk. It's even worse if it has been opened because you don't feel so guilty about dipping in!'

Nurses are classic 'comfort eaters', turning to chocolate for consolation when they feel tired, overworked and under stress... which is most of the time! No wonder so many have eating problems. Ironically, they are the very people who know the dangers of substituting chocolate for proper meals. Yet, because of the pressures of their job, they are extremely vulnerable to chocolate snack-attacks!'

When Janice joined the Chocoholic group, she weighed 10st 8lb and felt that the dreaded 11 stone barrier was looming: 'I have never touched 11 stone in my life,' she says. 'But I could see it coming!'

We put her on the Comfort Eaters programme, with strict instructions to look after herself with as much care and devotion as she looks after others. Her work involves seeing mothers through their pregnancies from the very beginning to several months after the birth, so she is a 'carer' in every sense of the word.

Here is an extract from a food diary she kept during the third week of her diet:

TUESDAY

Breakast 1oz unsweetened cereal, milk, 1 apple, 2 crisp-breads with a little low-fat spread. 'I have lost 4lb so far, which is great. I must keep this going. I am now allowed some chocolate, so I will save it for this afternoon after work.'

Lunch Sandwich of wholemeal bread, salad, tuna, lemon juice. 'This was satisfying. I am meeting mum after work. She is bound to want to go into Woolworths to buy some sweets. Will I be strong enough to stick to my allowance – which is 200 calories-worth daily?'

Snack 1 small banana. 'Felt very pleased with myself as I was able to pick out just a small Kit Kat and resisted the Pick-and-Mix sweet selection. I'll eat it later on, after my house calls are over.'

Supper Chicken casserole, mashed potato, fromage frais. 'This is easy. I had my Kit Kat at 5pm and I can still have a spritzer of white wine and soda and some fruit if I want it. I feel good.'

Janice was able to drop her chocolate allowance down to 150 calories daily without any problem, and is now nearly at her 'goal' weight. As you can see from the 'before' and 'after' pictures, she looks absolutely gorgeous. She says: 'The hardest part was having the discipline to think about my own meals, and to eat regularly.

'Most working mothers are so hard pushed that their own needs come way down the list. Believe me, it does make sense to get into a regular eating routine. You feel tons better and look better too. Everyone benefits, including your children and your husband.'

Name: **Betty Gower**
Age: 62   *Height*: 5ft 4in
Occupation: Office worker   *From*: New Eltham, London SE
Starting weight: **13st 3lb**   *Weight after 6 Weeks*: **12st 4lb**
Weight after 15 weeks: **12 stone**
Diet Plan: Weekend Indulger

Betty is a grandmother who lives alone but often entertains her growing grandchildren. She joined the Chocoholic group several months after our other guinea-pigs. She has always had a 'sweet tooth' and confessed that she uses her grandchildren as an 'excuse' to stock up with chocolate which she then consumes herself!

'I think most grannies like to give their grandchildren sweet treats – it's an expression of love which doesn't cost too much, and you are always guaranteed an enthusiastic reception from the children. My problem was that I was buying the chocolate early in the week and eating it before the children came on Saturday. When the scales registered 13st 3lb, I knew I had to do something. I saw a picture of myself at a party with a friend, looking huge in my flowered dress, which gave me quite a shock, too.'

We allowed Betty extra calories on Saturdays and Sundays to 'spend' on chocs, so long as she didn't buy her ration until Saturday morning. The first week, she lost a terrific 5lb, and then shed weight at the rate of two or three pounds a week. There was one small hiccup when she went away for the weekend and indulged in a few temptations. But, we later explained how to 'pre-think' your way through this kind of situation and deal with it. Now, she is able to control her chocoholism very well indeed.

Here is an extract from her food diary, after three weeks on the programme:

SUNDAY

Breakast 1 poached egg, 1 slice of wholemeal toast with low-fat spread. 'I will save my 300-calorie chocolate ration for this afternoon. It's in a tin, out of sight!'

Lunch Home-made vegetable soup with wholemeal toast and tomatoes, a few grapes. 'Will curl up with my chocs and a good book. Looking forward to it.'

Treat 1 small banana and half the chocolate allowance. 'Amazingly, I no longer feel that I must eat my chocolate quickly. I can enjoy it without guilt and I've even saved half to nibble in front of the TV.'

Supper Heinz Weight Watchers ready meal, green beans, broccoli, baked apple. 'Very satisfying and I still have some chocolate left. This is working well. I like the way I look in my clothes. My navy blue skirt is now feeling very roomy. It's great.'

Betty is now blooming. She aims to lose at least another stone, and is confident that she can keep her chocoholism under control. 'Learning to drop those guilt feelings is the most important part of the programme but even that doesn't work unless you eat all the food you are allowed. I must keep a food diary every week until I reach my goal. It is the only way to keep a check on myself, but worth it!'

Her 'pre-thinking' training has helped her cope with visits to friends and social occasions. Anyone can use this technique to help them plan their eating strategy in advance. All you have to do is to think through any eating situation before it happens and work out how you will handle it.

For instance, if you have to go away to stay with loving relatives (as Betty frequently does) who are bound to want to give you good food to eat, you should not be fearful that you will 'ruin' your diet. Be sensible – food is there to enjoy, not to fear. No one is going to make you stuff yourself silly with cakes and puddings. Your relatives will not be holding a gun to your head to make you take two helpings of their amazing dessert.

Just plan to enjoy each meal, eating slowly, and taking the things you want ... rather than everything you are offered. You will not be thought ungrateful if you refuse an extra roast potato or a slice of cake with your tea. You can always say that the food served up at mealtimes is so delicious that you don't want to spoil things by eating snacks. Plan to eat slowly, so no one notices if you don't eat everything on your plate. Offer to help clear away, so the food isn't left on the table too long. Be appreciative, but do not be bullied into eating more than you want. Offer to take the dog for a walk, or go to the shops for your hostess so you get plenty of exercise.

Betty says, 'It is amazing how much fitter I feel. Everyone has noticed ny new look. I have loads more energy and I don't feel that chocolate is ruling my life any more.'

CHAPTER EIGHT

MASSAGE, MEDITATION AND EXERCISE

While you are following your Chocoholic Diet, it is a good idea to increase the amount of exercise you take and to try out some do-it-yourself massage and meditation techniques.

MASSAGE

Our 'guinea-pigs' found the sensual pleasure of massage helped reduce their need for the sensual pleasure of eating chocolate. A long, delicious massage with essential oils has almost the same naughty, self-indulgent feeling as working your way through a box of Black Magic, with none of the calories! It made our slimmers relax, re-discover their bodies and enjoy being pampered. Moreover, chocolate cravings could be forestalled by a quick massage at the appropriate time. Tension often leads to irritability and tiredness which, in turn, can lead to a chocolate binge. So, dealing with tension by soothing away those aches and pains is obviously a good idea. Here are some techniques for you to try both at work and home:

At Work If you've had a really terrible day and the tea-time trolley (laden with chocolate bars, naturally) is about to appear, take time for a five-minute massage instead. If the boss objects, point out that Japanese workers usually have a masseuse on the staff.

1. Sit comfortably, with your bottom well back in your seat, feet apart and flat on the ground. If possible, place a small cushion in the hollow of your back. Now slowly raise your shoulders and drop them a few times, then circle your shoulders forwards and backwards, singly then together.

2. Now, place your right hand on your left shoulder and squeeze the tops of your shoulders with your fingers. Repeat with your left hand on your right shoulder.

3. Place the tips of your fingers on the back of your neck and, gently, massage each side of your vertebrae with your fingertips, stretching as far down your back as possible.

4. Place your thumbs under the back of your skull and spread your fingers out over your head. Press gently with your thumbs while rotating the balls of your fingers.

5. Place the tips of your middle fingers against the hollow each side of your brow-bone. Press gently, count six and relax.

6. Now move the same fingers to the top of your nose, placing them in the right-angled hollow made by your nose and brow-bone. Press upwards gently for a count of six, then relax.

(Nos. 5 and 6 are based on Japanese Shiatsu massage and are excellent for beating tension headaches and eyestrain.)

At home   You do not need a partner for this massage routine because all the movements can be performed by you. Try it when you are feeling low, or a bit lonely. Chocoholics who pig-out when partners are away working in the evening, could devote a little time to this massage and then curl up with a good book – *not* a box of chocs.

You will need some oils for the routine. It is easy to buy essential oils these days but they can be expensive. The best plan is to buy a large bottle of cheap massage oil (or use ordinary cooking oil) and add just a few drops of essential oil to the base.

If you are feeling particularly stressed, tense and anxious choose one of the following oils, or a combination of three: bergamot, geranium, lavender, camomile, ylang-ylang, neroli, rose and geranium. If you are very tired and want to be perked up (perhaps your partner is due home later), try rosemary or bergamot. If your sex life needs livening up, go for sandalwood, jasmine or patchouli.

You will also need a warm room with sufficient space to lie down, a towel, massage oil with appropriate essential oils added, and tissues.

1. Lie on your back and relax for a minute. Pour a little oil on your tummy and rub it in with circular movements.

2. Roll over. Press your fingertips on either side of your spine and rub gently. Bring your hands above shoulder level and rub your shoulder blades, neck and shoulders with gentle stroking movements.

3. Sit up slowly, take some more lotion and knead and press your legs. Work from the thighs towards the knees, then back again. Now do the same thing down to your ankles and back again.

4. Still sitting, press the tips of your thumbs either side of your spine. Press for a few seconds, relax and move your thumbs up about an inch (2.5cm). Repeat, working up as far as you can.

5. Stand up and knead and pinch your buttocks, then smooth on more oil in circular movements.

6. Now cover a chair with your towel and work some oil into your feet. The easiest way to do this is to rest one foot on the opposite thigh (like a modified 'half lotus' yoga position), and work really hard with fingers and thumbs all over the sole of your foot and between your toes. Repeat with the other foot.

7. Blot off the surplus oil with tissues, put on a bathrobe and rest on the bed for as long as you can. Set the alarm if you have an appointment as you may find that that you drop off to sleep.

MEDITATION

Although there is no evidence that meditation alone will cure chocoholism, it can definitely help you to control your life which, in turn, can only make it easier to kick the habit. It provides a valuable pause in the day when you can clear problems out of your mind and switch off completely. Afterwards, you feel refreshed and more able to cope. You do not have to meditate sitting on a carpet dressed in a loin cloth. On the contrary, you can do it anywhere. Try this simple routine at work or at home:

1. Take your shoes off. Now loosen any constricting clothes, particularly around your waist. Undo those overtight jeans, unzip that too-tight skirt. Close your eyes and sit comfortably with your hands in your lap or on your knees.

2. Breathe in and out slowly and gently. Now notice the contact of your body on the chair and your feet on the floor. Take a few comfortable breaths, imagining that you are taking in feelings of peace and tranquility and breathing out all the stresses and tensions and worries of the day.

3. Concentrate on your feet and make them relax, then work right up your body, concentrating on each bit and 'telling' it to relax completely. When you are perfectly relaxed, take a few deep, satisfying breaths and enjoy the gentle rhythm and flow of your own breathing. You will almost feel as though you are weightless and floating.

4. After a minute or two, bring your body back to life. First, be aware of the contact between your body and the chair, your feet and the floor. Next, bring your toes back to life by wiggling them. Stretch out your legs. Wiggle your

fingers, stetch your arms and hands. Give your whole body a really good stretch. Gently open your eyes. You'll feel terrific!

EXERCISE

Here are three different sets of exercises which can all be beneficial for chocoholics. The *first* is based on yoga, the ancient routine which really does help you revitalise your body and mind as well as unwind and relax. The *second* is a stretching routine, which will sort out all the aches and creaks of the day which could set you reaching for chocs. The *third* is a more energetic programme of movements which can be performed at home. This is designed to rev up your metabolism and should only be followed if you are less than 3 stone overweight and fairly fit. So do be sensible. If you have doubts about your ability to do any of the movements, check with your doctor.

1. YOGA
'Hatha' or physical yoga is a series of ancient postures or positions that move and improve almost every part of the human body. Do each movement very slowly, aiming for your best possible posture.

The Corpse This sounds deathly but it is a useful posture of deep relaxation which you should repeat before and after these exercises.

Lie on your back, legs apart, with feet flopping open. Your arms should be a little way away from your body, palms up, with fingers loosely curled. Now breath deeply and evenly for one minute.

The Cobra This is great for relieving tiredness and back pain and also helps sort out constipation and wind.

Lie, face down with your legs together, chin on the floor.

Place your forearms on the floor, elbows close to your body, hands by your shoulders. Lift your head, arch your back and pull your shoulders back and down. Look at the ceiling. Hold the position for a count of six, then bend your arms slowly and lower your body to the starting position. You should breathe out as you raise your body, breath in as you lower it. Repeat four times.

The Cat   If you have ever seen a cat stretch, you will understand why our feline friends are so supple. This exercise will strengthen your spine and tone up your tummy.

Go down on your hands and knees with your hands directly underneath your shoulders, fingers facing forwards. Slowly, let your back sink down, pushing your bottom up and out. Look up at the ceiling. Slowly, reverse the position by arching your back and pulling in your tummy. Drop your chin onto your chest. Hold for a count of five and repeat, then sit back on your heels for a few moments.

The Coil   If you have a wobbly bottom, this exercise is excellent. It tones the buttock muscles brilliantly. It also increases strength and mobility in the neck and helps flatten your tummy.

Lie on your back with your legs and feet together, toes pointed, and palms of your hands pressing downwards on the floor. Now bend your knees and bring them in as close to your chest as you can manage. Interlock your fingers and loop your hands over your knees. Pull your knees with your hands and raise your head towards them. Hold for a count of five, then lower your head to the floor and relax. Repeat twice and stretch out in the Corpse position (see page 98), for just a few seconds.

Salute to the Sun   This is a series of 12 movements which give a complete, all-round exercise in a very short time. It is ideal for early morning and really does set you up for the day. Try it once you have mastered the four basic exercises above.

The alternate stretching and bending helps improve circulation and aids breathing. Your digestion, tummy, back, arm and leg muscles are also given a boost. It is best to do this standing in loose clothes with bare feet on a soft rug. Try it once, then repeat if you have time:

1. Stand with your back straight, feet together. Press the palms of your hands together in front of your chest, with forearms horizontal and shoulders relaxed.

2. Now inhale, raising your arms above your head. Stretch upwards looking at the ceiling, tighten your buttocks and lean backwards, keeping your head and arms in a straight line.

3. Bend forward from your hips, exhaling as you do so. Tuck your head down to touch your knees and let your hands touch your legs. Now bend your knees so the palms of your hands touch the floor.

4. Look up, and take your left leg back as far as possible, with your knee on the floor. Your right knee should be bent, right heel on the floor. Arch your back.

5. Keeping your weight on your arms and hands, stetch your right leg back beside your left, so your legs, body and head make a straight line.

6. Now bend your arms and place your forehead, chest and knees on the floor. Breathe out and pull in your tummy. Breathe normally and take a mid-exercise rest for a few moments.

7. Push down on your hands, straightening your arms and arch your spine, lower your shoulders and look up. You are now in the Cobra pose, described above.

8. Raise your bottom into the air, straightening your legs and arms and letting your head hang down between them.

9. Transfer your weight onto your legs, lowering your heels.

10.   Bring your right foot forward, and place the sole on the floor. Lower your left knee, look up and inhale.

11.   Bring your left foot foreward next to the right one, straightening your legs, bend forward, clasp your legs and exhale.

12.   Now 'uncoil', raising your arms, body, and stretching so your arms are above your head. Slowly, go back to position 1.

2. STRETCHING EXERCISES

Do you ever arrive home from work feeling tired, hunched, and with nagging indigestion that won't go away? Before you reach for a drink, some medication or a comforting chocolate, go upstairs to your bedroom and do some very simple stretching exercises. They can help you unwind, internally as well as externally. You will find that those aches and creaks disappear and you feel full of life. Amazingly those hunger pangs (which weren't really hunger pangs at all) will have vanished.

Total Stretch   This is good for your back, legs, arms and tummy muscles and really does help you unwind. It is a great one to do if you've just driven home through congested traffic or arrived at your hotel after a long flight (leave the complientary chocolate on the pillow alone!).

Stand, feet together, arms above your head, fingers clasped loosely. Look up at your hands. Bend your knees and bring your hands down slowly to the horizontal position. Let your hands fall sideways and down, and relax your head forward. Pause, then reverse the movement. Repeat five times, breathing in as you raise your body, out as you lower it.

Leg and Arm Spine Stretch   This is super for legs, arms, tummy and posture. It is the one you often see athletes doing before a race, to help them warm up and prevent injury.

Stand straight, feet together, hands by your sides. Now take your left foot back, keeping your weight forward, left heel off the ground. Raise your right arm above your head. Raise your left leg and push your right arm back, keeping your right leg straight. Repeat five times with your left leg, right arm, then five times with your right arm, left leg.

Thigh and Hip Stretch   If you have been sitting down in a train or bus, or at work all day, this will help to sort out that cramped feeling in your bottom. It will also help slim your hips and thighs.

Sit on the floor, hands behind you for support, back straight, knees bent. Now swing your hips to the left, lowering both knees to touch the floor. Repeat to the right. Repeat the complete movement, right and left, five times.

Side and Waist Stretch   By improving your posture, you can appear much taller and slimmer. This exercise helps to whittle inches off your waistline and midriff and encourages you to sit and stand straight.

Stand with your feet about 2 feet (60cm) apart, hands by your sides. Now raise your right arm above your head, and bend your body, from the waist only, over to the left as far as you can go. Straighten up and repeat to the right. Repeat five times each side. After this mini work-out, you should be ready to tackle anything!

3. ENERGETIC EXERCISES
This routine is designed as a three-times weekly work out which will help rev up your metabolism. It is only suitable for slimmers who have 3 stone or less to lose and are reasonably fit. Do not attempt it if you are in bad shape. If in doubt, check with your doctor. Some lively music will help you stay the course!

Warm-up Start the routine by doing the Stretching Exercises above, repeating the Total Stretch exercise again at the end of the set.

Bent-Knee Sit Ups This is an excellent tummy-toner and the bent-knee position helps prevent back strain.

Lie on your back on the floor, with your feet on the floor, knees bent and legs slightly apart. Raise your arms to knee level, hands together, fingers straight. Leading with your head 'roll up' your back as far as you can to a sitting position, arms thrusting through your legs. Slowly, roll down, head last, until you are in the starting position. Repeat five to ten times, increasing repetitions as you improve.

Bottom and Hip Tightener If you hate your bottom, this is a superb exercise for you. But carry on dieting, too!

Kneel on the floor, placing your hands on the floor in front of you at shoulder level. Stretch your right leg out to one side, with the foot pointing forwards. Now raise the leg as high as you can keeping it at right angles to your body. Lower, repeat five times, then five times with the other leg. (To make this exercise slightly harder, and increase the work for your buttock and thigh muscles, do it with your knee bent, for the same number of repetitions.)

Thigh Lunge This is a controlled exercise which is harder than it sounds, but does great things for your thighs. Try not to wobble!

Stand with both feet on the floor, hands on your hips, with your right leg straight out in front, left leg behind, feet wide apart. Distribute your weight evenly between your feet. Now bend your right leg, moving your weight onto it. Keep your back straight and go down as low as you can without bending forward. Bend and straighten ten times. Swap legs and repeat.

Waist, Spine and Tummy Toner There are two separate movements in this exercise. It is fun and makes you feel very lively.

Stand with your feet apart, hands clasped above your head. Turn your body to the left, then lean forward from the waist, head down, arms straight out. Keep your head and arms in a straight line, and circle the upper part of your body down then up again, alternate ways. Repeat five times.

Now, lean forwards from the waist and thrust your hands through your legs, palms down, as far as is comfortably possible. Raise your body, place your hands on your waistline and lean back. Repeat five times.

Step Ups This is the original version of the popular 'stepping' routine which has taken off in a big way in health clubs and gyms. It is great for building up stamina.

Stand facing a small bench or the bottom step of the stairs. Now step up onto the bench with your left foot, bring your right foot up to meet it, then step down with your right foot, and bring your left foot down to meet it. Make sure you keep your back straight, your hands by your sides.

Running on the Spot End your workout with an 'indoor jog'. Run on the spot, with your back straight and your elbows bent. Do 50 paces, then relax.

CHAPTER NINE

HOW TO STAY SLIM AND EAT CHOCOLATE

So, you have reached your 'goal' weight and are wondering if you will be strong enough to stay in shape for good. This is the most important moment of your life. For, as every slimmer knows, it is far harder to keep weight off than to lose it in the first place. This is particularly true for chocoholics, who are exposed to their greatest temptation every single day.

Don't worry. I promise you that you can stay slim and enjoy a certain amount of chocolate without 'pigging-out' if you use the strategy outlined in this chapter.

FACE UP TO YOUR SUCCESS

The hardest task you face right now is to enjoy your achievement. Yes, amazing though it may seem, many slimmers find that reaching their target weight brings along a whole set of problems which they find difficult to cope with. Here are six examples, and how to tackle them:

1. *Coping with relationships* Your family or partner may feel threatened by the 'new' you. Suddenly, you are slim, dynamic and attractive, no longer plagued by the ups and downs of temperament that invariably accompany chocoholism. They are rattled, and may express this worry negatively, by being unreasonable, unhelpful or unloving. What you should do: be extra attentive but be firm in your determination to look good and do what you want to do. They

will soon adapt to the new you once they realise that the old you is still intact, too.

2. *Tackling challenges* When you were overweight it was very easy to use this as an excuse for opting out. You had a great reason for avoiding social events, work opportunities, sport, anything which might involve making an effort. Now, you no longer have that excuse. What you should do: dip one toe in the water at a time! Go to that party, book up that holiday, apply for that job – but don't do all three at once. Instead, revel in your new body by making the very best of your appearance. Invest in some new clothes, a good haircut, a night out. As soon as you realise that challenges are fun you will start to enjoy them instead of fearing them.

3. *Enjoying sex* For many chocoholics (especially Comfort Eaters and Romantics), chocs take the place of sex. Once your body is in great shape, there is no longer any reason for avoiding one of life's greatest pleasures. It is at this moment that you may realise that the sex-life you so carefully avoided wasn't all that great in the first place. Or, you may suddenly discover that there is no one to share your new-found sex-drive! What you should do: where there is an existing relationship which has gone sour, it is well worth trying to improve things. Your partner may be, quite rightly, fed up with your attitude and reluctant to get things going again. Some gentle wooing, romantic nights out and sexy underwear will work wonders. If not, counselling may be the answer. If you have avoided meeting the opposite sex and have no partner, it's a good idea to start being social again. Don't rush into a sexual relationship, though, until you have enjoyed some good old-fashioned romance first.

4. *Wish fulfilment* Many slimmers believe, erroneously, that being slim will make all their wildest dreams come true. Their partner will suddenly love them more, all their money worries will disappear, and they will suddenly enjoy a

Hollywood lifestyle. Sorry, but life isn't like that. True, being slim makes you feel better about yourself and more able to cope but it doesn't automatically make life rosier. Face this important fact head on and you will not be disappointed (and you will not reach for a box of chocs to cheer you up!).

5. *Size and power* Some overweight people sub-consciously enjoy the power that being fat brings. They like to be noticed and talked about. Men, particularly, are inclined to equate size with potency: the theory being that if their beer-belly is big it does not matter about other parts of their anatomy. If you suddenly miss being large, remember that fitness is macho too. You can always build up some muscle by working out.

6. *Dealing with jealousy* At first, it is lovely to be con-gratulated on your weight loss, but after a time you may realise that one or two of your closest friends are jealous of your success. They start making digs about your 'sunken cheeks' and 'thin legs', and follow up by dragging you into cafés for slices of chocolate cake and gâteau. Be strong. Recognise this as a sign of their insecurity, not yours. Deal with it by politely refusing their tempting offers. You *can* do it.

7. *Setting new targets* When you reach 'goal' there is always a moment of deflation because you no longer have the challenge ahead of hitting your target. Well, set another target – but this time make it to do with your home, work or fitness. Happiness is all about tackling new things and stretching yourself, so go for it!

HOW TO STAY IN CONTROL

There are ten important rules you must follow if you want to stay slim:

1. *Eat regularly* You must follow a sensible eating plan such as the one in this chapter if you are to keep your

chocoholism under control. That means having a meal or snack every few hours throughout the day. Do not ever let your blood sugar level get so low that you crave sweet foods.

2. *Be prepared* Every week, think about the various tasks you have to do and the appointments you have made. Plan your eating programme as well as your working and social programme.

3. *Take food with you* Never go anywhere without some fruit or a low-calorie snack in your shopping bag, briefcase or tool box. Don't be a sitting target for temptation.

4. *Keep busy* Pack plenty of activity into your life, so food takes second, third, or even fourth place. Re-decorate, go on bus rides, join local societies.

5. *Exercise regularly* Use the programme in Chapter Eight of this book to help you stay in amazing shape and rev up your metabolism.

6. *Have plenty of treats* You deserve the best. Allow yourself the sheer luxury of a half-day off to walk in the park, visit a gallery, curl up with a good book or simply stay in bed with your partner.

7. *Enjoy your meals and your chocolate allowance* You will see that your Maintenance Diet allows you plenty of food, including a generous ration of chocolate and choccy dishes. Please eat them up and enjoy them.

8. *Keep your body image strong* Every day, look at yourself in the mirror and make a point of enjoying what you see. Vanity is healthy. Take time out to visualise yourself in future situations like a family party, wedding, or holiday, looking fit, well, and slim. Imagine every detail, from what you are wearing, to the food you are eating and the company you are in.

9. *Relax* Stress is a diet killer. Beat it by taking short, inexpensive breaks whenever possible. Psychologists say that

they are better for you than a long, annual holiday which can be stressful in itself.

10. *Weigh yourself weekly* It is crazy to weigh in more often than that because fluid changes in the body can play havoc with your 'official' weight. Instead, step on the scales once a week, at the same time of day, wearing the same clothes. Allow yourself a 5lb 'ceiling' above your goal weight. If you go above that level, go back on your Chocoholic Diet for a week or so. Even if you slip back, don't panic. Slimming may be a lifetime's occupation, but it is fun, too.

CHOCS AROUND THE WORLD

Once you have managed to lose weight and control your chocoholism, you can start enjoying it. The best way to eat chocolate is in small amounts, savouring every little bit. It is easier to eat less when you pay more, so indulge yourself with expensive chocolate once in a while. Here is a guide to some of the best places to buy 'posh' chocolate:

London, England Leonidas, the famous Belgian choc-olatiers, have a shop on the ground floor at Selfridges with a selection of delicious hand-made luxury chocs. Charbonnet and Walker in Bond Street is the shop for the real connoisseur but don't visit it if you are strapped for cash.

Paris, France Try Maisons du Chocolat for amazing centres, incredible truffles and gorgeous slab chocolate.

Geneva, Switzerland Jenny's at the railway station is the best shop but amazing chocs are everywhere.

Zurich, Switzerland Sprungli or Teuscher sell the sensational Pfister chocolates – every mouthful is orgasmic!

Brussels, Belgium   Any branch of Leonidas or Godiva is a chocoholic's paradise.

Aspen, USA   At the Rocky Mountain Chocolate Factory the chocolate is made right in the shop window, so it is almost impossible not to go in and taste it. They sell huge slabs but it is much safer to buy the smaller bars.

Hong Kong   If you stay at the Hilton, try the Gerard Dubois chocs – lovely.

Copenhagen, Denmark   Try the help-yourself chocolate bar at the Airport but do eat a protein-packed snack first.

Hamburg, Germany   Go to the Condi Café in the Vier Jahreszeitsen, where they make their own, yummy chocs.

Vienna, Austria   Look for the Kuvkonditorei Oberlaa branches where they sell chocolates made by master chocolatier, Karl Shuhmacher.

Best chocs by aeroplane   Chocoholic travellers recommend the Lufthansa selection because their after-dinner chocolates are hand-made by small manufacturers.

YOUR MAINTENANCE DIET

Here is the diet which will help you stay slim. It allows about 1500 calories for women, and 2000 for men. Follow it for two weeks after you reach your target weight. If you are still losing, increase your calories by 100 each week, choosing items from the list at the end of this chapter (sorry, this does not include chocolate) until you maintain a steady weight.

Women can also have 150 calories daily of chocolate (including bars, sweets, individual chocs, biscuits or dishes chosen from the recipes in Chapter Ten), men can have 200 calories. This can be eaten in two or three 'lumps' during the week but not all at one go. Avoid buying it all at once, and make sure you really enjoy every mouthful.

In France, chocolate connoisseurs (mostly very slim people!) like to take their daily treat of dark, delicious, expensive chocolate with a glass of wine or cognac. Since you are allowed a daily alcohol ration, there is no reason why you shouldn't do the same. One of our successful chocoholic slimmers now has a very expensive chocolate wafer mint in bed every night, plus a small brandy while she watches an erotic video. This is on the nights when her husband is away working. When he's home, they only manage to watch about 20 minutes of the video!

DAILY ALLOWANCES

You may have ½ pint (275ml) skimmed milk for your tea and coffee, plus unlimited water and mineral water. Go easy on the caffeine, and try to include more water and herbal drinks in your diet. Camomile, lemon and tropical fruit teas are all delicious. Although diet soft drinks contain very few calories and most eating programmes allow them, do take it easy. Unfortunately, too many of these sweet-tasting drinks could have a nasty effect on your taste-buds and turn you into a chocolate junkie again. Beware!

You can also have unlimited vegetables from the list on page 47. Serve them imaginatively, as salads with lemon juice, herbs and vinegar dressings, or lightly boiled, steamed or stir fried in very little oil. Pile them up on your plate at every meal so you never feel deprived.

MALE EXTRAS Choose *one* each day.

- 2 large slices of wholemeal bread with a little low-fat spread
- 1 pint beer or lager

- 6oz (120g) mashed potato made with skimmed milk
- 2oz (50g) any lean meat

ALCOHOL ALLOWANCE   Choose *one* each day.
- ½ pint beer or lager
- 1 glass dry wine
- 2 pub measure 'short' drinks with low-calorie mixers only.

Non-drinkers can have an extra slice of bread or a small wholemeal roll.

EVERY DAY   Eat *one* Breakfast, *one* Light Meal, *one* Supper and *one* Metabolic Boosting High Protein Snack which you should eat when you feel that your energy is flagging and your taste-buds are tingling.

BREAKFASTS
- 1 rasher well-grilled back bacon, grilled tomatoes, 1 slice wholemeal toast, 1 apple
- Sandwich of 2 slices wholemeal bread with one of these fillings:
  - 1 small banana
  - 1 rasher well-grilled streaky bacon and tomatoes
  - ½oz (12g) grated low-fat Cheddar cheese
- 1oz any unsweetened cereal, with milk from allowance, 1 size 3 egg, 2 crispbreads with a little low-fat spread
- 1 carton low-calorie yogurt, any flavour, 1 slice wholemeal toast topped with a little Marmite or 1 tsp jam or marmalade, 4fl oz (100ml) unsweetened fruit juice
- Breakfast milkshake made by blending together ¼ pint (125ml) skimmed milk (extra to allowance), 1 large chopped banana, 1 carton low-calorie banana yogurt, sprinkling of cocoa powder

LIGHT MEALS

Jacket Potatoes   10oz (250g) jacket potato with salad and vegetables from 'free' list and one of these fillings:

- 2 tbsp baked beans and ½oz (12g) grated Edam cheese
- 1 carton Shape coleslaw
- 2 tbsp natural yogurt mixed with a little horseradish sauce and 1oz (25g) chopped chicken or ham (no skin or fat)
- 1 small can tuna-in-brine, mashed with lemon juice

OR Choose your Jacket Potato meal from a takeaway such as Spud-U-Like where you may choose any of these fillings: baked beans, cottage cheese with chives, Mexican Bean salad, Spring Salad or Sweetcorn.

Meals on Toast   2 slices wholemeal toast topped with one of the following plus 1 apple, orange, pear or small banana:

- 1 poached egg and 2 tbsp baked beans or canned spaghetti in tomato sauce
- 1 tin tuna-in-in brine topped with ½oz (12g) grated Edam cheese
- grilled tomatoes topped with 1 rasher well-grilled back bacon
- 2oz (50g) mushrooms poached in chicken stock, mixed with 1oz lean chopped ham

Meals with a Chocolate Recipe

- 8oz (250g) chicken leg, no skin, huge mixed salad, 1 portion Chocolate Banana Cake (*see* recipe, page 121)
- Chocolate Banana Sandwich (*see* recipe, page 135), 1 apple
- 6oz (150g) any grilled fish, grilled tomatoes and salad from the 'free' list, Chocolate Mousse (*see* recipe, page 128), 1 apple, a few grapes

Salads   Large mixed salad from 'free' list with lemon juice or vinegar and herb dressing with one of the following:

- 10oz (250g) chicken wing, skin removed, 1 small wholemeal roll with a little low-fat spread, 1 large banana or 2 apples or pears

- Small piece quiche (cheese, meat or fish), 1 apple, orange, or small banana or low-calorie yogurt
- 4oz (100g) smoked fish, 1 slice wholemeal bread with a little low-fat spread, slice of lemon, a few grapes

Sandwiches 2 slices wholemeal bread with salad from 'free' list and one of these fillings and accompaniments:

- 1oz (25g) chicken, ham or any lean meat without fat or skin, 1 apple, pear or small banana

MAIN MEALS

Cold Meals Large mixed salad from the 'free' list with one of the following:

- 2oz (50g) any cold, lean meat, 1 wholemeal roll with a little low-fat spread, 1oz (25g) Edam or low-fat Cheddar cheese
- 1 medium slice quiche, 2 tbsp sweetcorn, 1 apple
- 1 pack Heinz Weight Watchers Pasta Plus Pasta Shells with Vegetables and Prawns, served cold, 1 slice wholemeal bread with a little low-fat spread, 1 large banana

Hot Meals

- 3oz (75g) pasta (dry weight) topped with one of the following:
- tinned tomatoes with 4oz (100g) shelled prawns, garlic, herbs, large mixed salad; 1oz (25g) scoop vanilla icecream with 1 portion Chocolate Sauce (*see* recipe, page 133) *OR* 1 small wholemeal roll with ½oz (12g) Camembert or other soft cheese
- 5oz (125g) lean lamb or pork chop, grilled, thin gravy, large portion 'free' vegetables, 3oz (75g) mashed potato (use skimmed milk from allowance for mashing), baked apple with 1 tbsp yogurt
- 5oz (125g) lean rump or fillet steak, grilled, 3oz (75g) oven chips, grilled tomatoes, watercress, large mixed salad and vegetables from the 'free' list

- 1 large slice of melon or ½ grapefruit with ginger and/or artificial sweetener, 3½oz (87g) gammon steak, grilled, 2 tbsp peas, 1 slice pineapple, canned in juice, 6oz (150g) jacket potato, large portion salad and 'free' vegetables
- 4oz (100g) calves' liver, grilled, 1 rasher well-grilled back bacon, grilled tomatoes, vegetables from the 'free' list, 1 portion Chocolate and Raisin Rice Pudding (*see* recipe, page 132) or Chocolate Coconut Icecream (*see* recipe, page 126)
- Casserole of 4oz (100g) lean stewing beef cooked in 1 can low-calorie tomato soup with sliced onions, 2tbsp sliced carrots, herbs, garlic and beef stock, vegetables from the 'free' list, 1 large banana

Vegetarian Meals
- 2 Bird's Eye vegetable burgers, grilled, grilled tomatoes, 3oz (75g) oven chips, large mixed salad from the 'free' list, 2 tbsp peas, 1oz (25g) scoop vanilla icecream with 1 portion Chocolate Sauce (*see* recipe, page 133)
- Sainsbury's Broccoli Provençal or St Michael's Vegetable Chilli with additional vegetables and salad from the 'free' list and ½oz (12g) grated low-fat Cheddar cheese

Eating out
Choose melon or clear soup as a starter and then go for lean meat or fish (no sauces) and a good selection of vegetables. At Indian restaurants, choose Chicken Tikka or Tandoori with plain boiled rice and salad. Chinese restaurants are more difficult. Your best bet is a Chicken Chop Suey with plain boiled rice. Avoid all fatty foods, those with creamy sauces, and the sweet trolley unless you are feeling very strong indeed. If you do go 'over the top', make up for it by cutting out your alcohol and chocolate allowance for a couple of days.

Metabolic Boosting High Protein Snacks

Choose *one* each day. Make sure you have your snack with you – most of these are easy to pack:

- 2 crispbreads with scraping of Marmite and 1 small carton cottage cheese
- 2 sticks celery, filled with 1 heaped dsp peanut butter
- 2oz (50g) thin ham, spread with 1oz (25g) Philadelphia Light spread, rolled up and cut into bite-sized pieces
- 3 Matthews Mini Kievs with grilled tomatoes
- 1oz (25g) Edam cheese on a skewer with chopped green peppers, tomatoes, mushrooms, 2 crispbreads with scraping of low-fat spread
- 1 slice Nimble bread, 1 cold fish finger and salad
- 2oz (50g) John West prawns, drained, 3oz (75g) boiled rice, onion, 1 tsp peas, 1 tsp diced carrot
- 1 mug Batchelors Slim a Soup Special Tomato and Vegetable with Croutons topped with ½oz (12g) grated low-fat Cheddar
- 1oz (25g) Edam cheese, 1 apple

100 CALORIE EXTRAS (If you are still losing weight 2 weeks after reaching your target weight add one of these each day for a week. If you are still losing add another, and so on.)

- 1 slice wholemeal bread or small wholemeal roll with a little low-fat spread
- 3oz (75g) potato, mashed with skimmed milk
- 3oz (75g) any pasta (dry weight)
- 2oz (50g) chicken (no skin) or lean ham
- 1 large banana or 2 medium apples, oranges or pears
- 2tbsp sweetcorn and 3tbsp peas or carrots
- 1 low-fat pork sausage

CHAPTER TEN

CHOC FULL OF TASTE!

Here is a selection of choccy recipes which have been cut down to the minimum calories, especially for chocoholics. You may include them in your diet as part of your daily chocolate calorie allowance only. For instance, if you are on one of the programmes that alows 200 calories of chocolate each day, you can either choose that from the chocolate list (page 140) *or* from the recipes given here. Not both, sorry!

Don't forget, these dishes are to enjoy. Don't feel guilty about savouring every single mouthful. A word of warning: if you are cooking up something just for yourself and the ingredients are given for four people, you could be in trouble. It is safer to divide the ingredients into four and make just one portion, invite three hungry people around to share the meal, or make up four portions and hide three in the fridge or a cake tin with a lid! For biscuit recipes, it is essential to store the goodies in a tin or make them only for special occasions when you are expecting a hoard of hungry guests. No cheating, please!

N.B. The ingredients in the recipes have been given in ounces and the nearst equivalent measurement in grams. A set of kitchen scales aids accurate weighing of the solid ingredients and a graduated jug (1 pint/575ml) for liquids. Spoon measurements are level. You should work in either imperial weights or metric but not both.

APHRODISIAC DISHES

These are mouthwatering, fun-shaped treats for lovers. Don't forget, the more real love and affection you have, the less likely you are to be zapped by the 'false' kind, conjured up by the phenylethylamine in chocolate.

Use these recipes to seduce the important person, or people, in your life and yourself (and don't forget to count the calories as part of your daily chocolate allowance)!

CHOCOLATE ALMOND NIBBLES

2oz (50g) self-raising flour
½ level tsp (2.5 ml) baking powder
1oz (25g) cocoa powder
1oz (25g) almonds, blanched and chopped
5oz (150g) soft brown sugar
orange rind of ½ orange
2oz (50g) butter
3oz (75g) Shape soft cheese
2 large eggs

1. Sieve together the flour, baking powder and cocoa.
2. Add the almonds, sugar and orange rind. Beat the butter and cheese together.
3. Beat into the dry ingredients and then add the eggs, mixing thoroughly.
4. Spoon into a greased 7-inch (18cm) cake tin and level the top. Bake for 50 minutes at 160°C, 325°F, Gas 3, until cooked.
5. Cool on a wire rack, and cut into 16 squares. Store them out of sight in a tin until needed.

Makes 16 pieces   *80 calories per piece*

CHOUX BOOBS

Pastry   ¼ pint (150ml) water
2oz (50g) low-fat spread for cooking

2½oz (70g) plain flour, sieved
pinch of salt
2 large eggs, lightly beaten
Filling   16 level tbsp (240ml) chocolate icecream
8oz (25g) sliced strawberries or raspberries
Topping   8tsps (40ml) strawberry jam
8 chocolate buttons

1.   Place water and spread in a small saucepan and bring to the boil over a moderate heat.

2.   Remove from the heat and immediately add the sieved flour and salt. Beat with a wooden spoon until mixture leaves the sides of the pan. Cool slightly.

3.   Beat the eggs in small quantities into the cooled mixture.

4.   Place 8tbsp (120ml) of the mixture on a baking sheet lined with non-stick baking paper.

5.   Bake near the top of a pre-heated oven 220°C, 425°F, Gas 7 for 20 minutes. Reduce the temperature to 190°C, 375°F, Gas 5 and cook for another 10 minutes.

6.   Slit base of buns to allow steam to escape and then cool.

7.   When cold, fill the buns with icecream and fruit.

8.   Top with jam and a single chocolate button.

Serves 6   *160 calories per portion*

CHOC PEAKS

2oz (50g) rolled oats
3tbsp (45ml) whisky
1tsp (5ml) clear honey
juice of 1 lemon
8oz (225g) low-fat cottage cheese, sieved
5fl oz (150ml) carton low-fat yogurt, chilled
2oz (50g) stoned dates, chopped
½ oz (15g) dark chocolate for decoration

1.   Spread the oats on a baking tray and toast lightly under the grill.

2.   Place the whisky, honey and lemon juice in a small bowl and stir.

3.   Place the cottage cheese and yogurt in a large bowl and gradually beat in the whisky mixture, dates and most of the oats.

4.   Divide between four serving dishes and decorate with a few oats. Chill and sprinkle with grated chocolate just before serving.

Serves 4   *170 calories per portion*

CHOCOLATE WOBBLY BITS   *(Microwave recipe)*

2tbsp (30 ml) cornflour
1tbsp (15ml) cocoa powder
1tbsp (15ml) Fructose
½ pint (275ml) skimmed milk
4tsp (1.25ml) vanilla essence
1tsp (5ml) low-fat spread
strips of orange to decorate

1.   Blend cornflour, cocoa and Fructose together in a large jug.

2.   Gradually stir in the milk.

3.   Cook on maximum, uncovered, for 1 minute. Stir well and then cook on maximum for a further 30 seconds or until the mixture thickens.

3.   Stir again, then add the low-fat spread and vanilla essence.

4.   Pour into individual dishes, cover with clingfilm and leave to set.

5.   Decorate with orange strips before serving.

Serves 2   *125 calories per portion*

CAKES AND BISCUITS

Once you have trained your palate to accept smaller quantities of chocolate, it is safe to indulge in these. A word of warning however: make your cakes and biscuits in small batches only and store them, out of sight, in an airtight container.

CHOCOLATE BANANA CAKE

½oz (15g) cocoa
3½oz (90g) wholemeal self-raising flour
1 level tsp (5ml) baking powder
2oz (50g) walnuts
4oz (100g) margarine
5 level tbsp (75ml) Hermesetas Sprinkle Sweet
1 large ripe banana
2 eggs, size 2

1. Sieve together the cocoa, flour and baking powder.
2. Chop the walnuts.
3. Cream together the margarine and Sprinkle Sweet.
4. Mash the banana and beat into the creamed mixture.
5. Lightly beat the eggs and mix them into the creamed mixture a little at a time.
6. Stir in the flour mixture and walnuts.
7. Turn into a greased and lined 7-inch (18cm) square shallow tin. Bake in a preheated oven at 180°C, 350°F, Gas 4 for 30 minutes. Cool on a wire rack.

Makes 16 squares   *110 calories per portion*

CHOC CHIP COOKIES

8oz (225g) self-raising flour
pinch of salt
5oz (150g) sunflower margarine

4oz (100g) caster sugar
2oz (50g) plain chocolate chips
1 egg, size 3, beaten

1. Sift the flour and add the salt. Rub in the margarine until the mixture resembles breadcrumbs.
2. Add the sugar and the chocolate chips.
3. Next add the egg and mix to a firm dough.
4. Knead gently on a floured surface until smooth.
5. Place inside a plastic bag and chill for 30 minutes.
6. Roll the dough out thinly, and using a 2-inch (5cm) cutter, cut out 30 biscuits.
7. Place on a lightly greased baking sheet and prick all over with a fork.
8. Bake for 12-15 minutes at 180°C, 350°F, Gas 4.
9. Allow to cool on a baking sheet.

Makes 30 biscuits *90 calories per cookie*

CAROB DISHES

Most chocoholics find it difficult to enjoy the taste of carob in 'pretend' chocolate bars. However, this well-known chocolate substitute is more palatable when used in cooking especially if it is combined with fruit. It also has the advantage of having none of the side-effects of chocolate, so the urge to eat more than is good for you is not so compelling.

It is worth trying these recipes. Carob is available from most health food shops.

CAROB BLACK FOREST GATEAU

3 eggs, size 3, separated
3oz (85g) caster sugar
2½oz (70g) plain white flour
½oz (15g) carob powder

6oz (175g) black cherries, canned in natural juice, stoned
5oz (150g) Shape Double

1.   Whisk the egg whites and sugar together until thick and foamy.

2.   Mix the flour and carob powder together. Gently, fold into the whites, and pour into 2 loose-bottomed, lightly oiled and lined 8-inch (20cm) cake tins.

3.   Bake at 180°C, 350°F, Gas 4 for 15-20 minutes until springy to the touch. Allow to cool on a wire rack.

4.   Chop the cherries. Whisk the cream into soft peaks and fold into the fruit. Sandwich the sponge together with the mixture, reserving some to decorate the top.

Serves 8   *160 calories per portion*

CAROB MOUSSE

3½oz (90g) Plamil carob bar
grated rind and juice of ½ small orange
2 eggs, size 2, separated
1 tsp (5ml) powdered gelatine
fine strips of orange rind, for decoration

1.   Place the carob in a small bowl over a pan of simmering water and stir until melted.

2.   Remove from heat and stir in the grated orange rind and beat in the egg yolks.

3.   Place the orange juice in another small basin and sprinkle on the gelatine. Leave to stand for 5 minutes. Place the basin in a pan containing a little simmering water and leave until the gelatine has dissolved.

4.   Stir into the carob mixture.

5.   Whisk the egg whites to form stiff peaks and fold into the mixture.

6.   Divide between 4 individual serving dishes. Chill in the

refrigerator until set. Decorate with strips of orange rind.

Serves 4   *180 calories per portion*

ORANGE CAROB CAKE

3oz (75g) low-fat cooking margarine
8oz (225g) self-raising flour
4tbsp (60ml) Hermesetas Sprinkle Sweet
4oz (100g) Plamil carob bar, chopped
grated rind and juice of 1 orange
a little skimmed milk
1 egg, size 3

1.   Preheat the oven to 180°C, 350°F, Gas 4. Line and brush a 2lb loaf tin lightly with oil.
2.   Rub the margarine into the flour in a mixing bowl.
3.   Add the Sprinkle Sweet, orange rind and carob. Stir lightly.
4.   Squeeze the orange and pour the juice into a measuring jug.
5.   Add enough milk to make the liquid up to ¼ pint (150ml).
6.   Beat the egg and pour into the dry ingredients. Add the orange juice and milk mixture, stir and turn into the loaf tin.
7.   Bake for about 1 hour or until an inserted skewer comes out clean. Cool, then turn out on a wire rack. Serve in slices.

Serves 6   *160 calories per portion*

DRINKS

Here are some great recipes for long, delicious chocolate drinks. They are very tasty but not too high in calories. Sip them slowly, enjoying the full flavour of the chocolate and their scrumptious ingredients.

CARIBBEAN MILKSHAKE

1 pint (575ml) skimmed milk
2-3 level tsps (10-15ml) drinking chocolate
5oz (150g) tub natural, low-fat yogurt
1 banana, cut into three pieces
1 tbsp (15ml) rum (optional)
1 level tsp (5ml) chopped nuts to decorate

1. Place all the ingredients in a blender and mix until smooth.
2. Divide between 4 glasses and decorate with nuts.

Serves 4   *110 calories per glass*

CHOCOLATE MINT MILKSHAKE

10fl oz (272ml) skimmed milk
1 tbsp (15ml) drinking chocolate powder
2-3 drops peppermint essence
3 ice cubes
Hermesetas Sprinkle Sweet to taste

1. Place all ingredients in a liquidiser and blend for 30 seconds.
2. Pour into a tall glass and drink slowly!

Serves 1   *130 calories per glass*

FROZEN DESSERTS

Frozen desserts and icecream are easy to make at home and safer for slimmers than the shop-bought kind because it is easier to control the calories. These are good for dinner parties or pure self-indulgence.

CHOCOLATE COCONUT ICECREAM

¼ pint (150ml) semi-skimmed milk
2oz (50g) dessicated coconut
1 level tbsp (15ml) cocoa
2 level tbsp (30ml) Hermesetas Sprinkle Sweet
1 level tsp (5ml) gelatine
2 tbsp (30ml) water
¼ pint (150ml) whipping cream
¼ pint (150ml) half-fat evaporated milk
2 tbsp (30ml) Malibu

1.   Place the milk, coconut and cocoa in a small pan and heat until boiling, stirring all the time.
2.   Turn into a basin and stir in the Sprinkle Sweet.
3.   Dissolve the gelatine in the water and add to the milk mixture. Leave until cold but not set.
4.   Whip the cream until it forms soft peaks. Whip the evaporated milk until it is light and fluffy.
5.   Fold the cream and evaporated milk into the milk mixture with the Malibu.
6.   Turn into a plastic container and freeze for 2 hours.
7.   Turn into a chilled bowl and whisk to break down the ice crystals. Return to the container and freeze until solid.

Serves 8   *160 calories per portion*

CHOCOLATE AND MINT ICECREAM

¼ pint (150ml) natural low fat yogurt
5oz (150g) skimmed-milk soft cheese
peppermint flavouring
green food colouring (optional)
3tbsp (45ml) Hermesetas Sprinkle Sweet
2 egg whites
½oz (15g) plain chocolate drops

1. Gradually beat the yogurt into the cheese then whisk together until light.
2. Whisk in a few drops of peppermint flavouring, food colouring if desired, and the Hermesetas Sprinkle Sweet.
3. Spoon the mixture into a shallow metal container and cover. Place in the freezer and leave for one hour.
4. Empty into a chilled bowl and whisk using a mixer to break down the ice crystals.
5. Freeze for another 30 minutes and repeat the whisking process.
6. Whisk the egg whites until stiff but not dry.
7. Carefully fold in the egg whites and the chocolate drops, return the mixture to the freezer container and freeze.
8. 30 minutes before serving, remove from the freezer and place in the fridge.

Serves 6   *55 calories per portion*

PUDDINGS (COLD)

There is nothing like a chilly choccy pudding to tickle your taste buds at the end of a meal. These are all quick to prepare so save some calories for them from your daily allowance.

CHOCCY CHESTNUT MOUSSE

½ pint (275ml) skimmed milk
3 level tbsp (45ml) cocoa
sweetener
6oz (175g) chestnut purée
2 tbsp (30ml) hot water
1 sachet (10g) gelatine
2 egg whites

1. Heat ¼ pint (150ml) milk to boiling point.
2. Mix cocoa to a paste with some of the remaining milk.

3.   Blend the hot milk with the cocoa and then place back in the pan and bring to the boil.

4.   Remove from the heat and cool slightly.

5.   Add sweetener to taste.

6.   Place in a blender with the chestnut purée and the rest of the milk, and mix until smooth.

7.   Dissolve the gelatine in the hot water and add to the blender. Mix again.

8.   Place in a bowl and refrigerate until the mousse just starts to set.

9.   Whisk the egg whites until stiff but not dry. Fold into the chocolate mixture.

10.   Divide between 4 individual serving dishes and chill.

Serves 4   *165 calories per portion*

CHOCOLATE MINTY MERINGUES

1oz (25g) Mint Matchmakers, broken into small pieces
4oz (100g) mint choc icecream
4 meringue nests
4tbsp (60ml) Cadbury's Chocolate Liqueur
chocolate, for decoration

1.   Fold the broken Matchmakers into the icecream.

2.   Spoon a portion into each meringue nest.

3.   Sprinkle with liqueur and decorate with a *small* amount of chocolate.

Serves 4   *205 calories per portion*

CHOCOLATE MOUSSE

1 carton (7.7oz/215g) Carnation Light unsweetened condensed semi-skimmed milk (or tin)
2 level tsp (10ml) powdered gelatine
4tbsp (60ml) water

1 sachet Ovaltine Options Choc-n-Orange or Choc-O-lait
mandarin segments to decorate

1.   Chill the carton of Carnation Light overnight
2.   Sprinkle the gelatine onto 2tbsp (30ml) of cold water in
a cup. Leave to soak for 5 minutes.
3.   Stand the cup in a pan containing a little simmering
water and leave until the gelatine is dissolved or microwave
on Defrost for 30 seconds.
4.   Mix the Ovaltine Options with 2tbsp (30ml) hot water to
make a smooth paste.
5.   Whip the Carnation Light until very frothy. Continue
whipping while adding the dissolved gelatine and chocolate
mixture.
6.   Turn into a serving dish or 4 individual dishes and chill
until set. Decorate with mandarin segments.

Serves 4   *80 calories per portion*

CHOCOLATE PEAR TRIFLE

3 trifle sponges
3 level tsps (15ml) reduced-sugar jam
15oz (425g) can pears in juice
2 tbsp (30ml) cherry brandy
8fl oz (225ml) orange juice
10fl oz (275ml) water
1 sachet (10g) gelatine
3 level tbsp (45ml) Hermesetas Sprinkle Sweet
3 level tbsp (45ml) custard powder
1 level tbsp (15ml) cocoa
¾ pint (425ml) semi-skimmed milk
1oz (25g) flaked almonds

1.   Split the trifle sponges and fill with jam. Place in a glass
bowl.

2.   Drain the pears and reserve the juice. Mix 2 tbsp (30ml) juice with the cherry brandy and sprinkle over the sponges.

3.   Mix the remaining juice with the orange juice and make up to 1 pint (575ml) with water.

4.   Dissolve the gelatine in the juice and add 1 level tbsp (15ml) Sprinkle Sweet. Pour over the sponges and chill until set.

5.   Mix the custard powder and cocoa with a little milk until smooth.

6.   Heat the remaining milk until almost boiling and then add to the custard mixture, stirring continuously. Return to the pan and bring to the boil while stirring. Simmer for 2 minutes.

7.   Pour into a cool basin and add the remaining Sprinkle Sweet. Leave to cool, whisking lightly very frequently.

8.   Pour over the jelly. Toast the almonds and sprinkle on top.

Serves 6   *180 calories per portion.*

CHOCOLATE POTS WITH COINTREAU

2 eggs, size 3
2 level tbsp (30ml) cocoa
¾ pint (425ml) skimmed milk
2tbsp (30ml) Cointreau
Hermesetas Sprinkle Sweet, to taste
orange peel
4 squirts of Anchor Light Aerosol cream to decorate

1.   Whisk the eggs with the cocoa powder in a bowl.

2.   Heat the milk almost to boiling point and gradually add to the egg mixture stirring all the time.

3.   Set the bowl over a pan of simmering water and cook stirring constantly until the mixture thickens.

4.   Strain into ramekin dishes and stand in a deep roasting tin.

5.   Pour hot water into the roasting tin to come halfway up the sides of the ramekins.

6.   Cover with greaseproof paper and bake in the oven at 170°C, 325°F, Gas 3 for 25-30 minutes or until just set.

7.   Allow to cool and serve decorated with a squirt of Anchor Light aerosol cream and a thin strip of orange peel.

Serves 4   *155 calories per portion*

PUDDINGS (HOT)

Centuries ago, chocolate was served hot as a rather bitter-tasting drink. The cocoa flavour develops a smoothness and richness when hot and, these days, you can add a sweet taste without too many extra calories by using a sugar substitute.

CHOCOLATE AND CHERRY STEAMED PUDDING

3oz (75g) margarine
4 level tbsp (60ml) Hermesetas Sprinkle Sweet
2 eggs, size 2
5oz (150g) self-raising flour
½oz (15g) cocoa
½ level tsp (2.5ml) baking powder
4 tbsp (60ml) semi-skimmed milk
3oz (75g) glacé cherries

1.   Cream the margarine and Sprinkle Sweet together.

2.   Lightly beat the eggs and then add to the creamed mixture a little at a time, beating well after each addition.

3.   Sieve together the flour, cocoa and baking powder and then add to the mixture with the milk and cherries.

4.   Turn into a greased basin and cover with greaseproof paper and foil. Steam for 1½ hours. Serve with chocolate sauce (*see* recipe on page 133).

CHOCOLATE AND RAISIN RICE PUDDING

1½oz (40g) pudding rice
3 level tbsp (45ml) Hermesetas Sprinkle Sweet
2oz (50g) raisins
2 level tsp (10ml) cocoa
1 pint (575ml) semi-skimmed milk

1. Place the rice, Sprinkle Sweet and raisins in an oven-proof dish.
2. Mix the cocoa with a little of the milk until smooth.
3. Add the remaining milk and pour over the rice.
4. Bake at 150°C, 300°F, Gas 2 for about 2 hours. Stir after ½ hour and again after 1 hour.

Serves 4   *150 calories per portion*

CHOCOLATE BAKED CUSTARD

4oz (100g) fresh white breadcrumbs
1 pint (575ml) skimmed milk
3 level tbsp (45ml) cocoa
Hermesetas Sprinkle Sweet
1 egg, size 3, lightly beaten

1. Place the breadcrumbs in a 1½pint (850ml) ovenproof dish.
2. Blend 2tbsp (30ml) of the skimmed milk with the cocoa until smooth.
3. Gradually stir in the remaining milk and pour into a saucepan and bring to the boil.
4. Add Sprinkle Sweet to taste.
5. Pour the cocoa mixture over the egg, stirring all the time and then strain over the breadcrumbs.
6. Leave to stand for 20 minutes and then bake for 45-50

minutes at 180°C, 350°F, Gas 4.

Serves 4   *160 calories per portion*

CHOCOLATE FONDUE   *(Microwave recipe)*
fresh fruit, cut into chunks or strips
4oz (100g) plain chocolate drops
½ pint (275ml) Shape Single
¼ pint (150ml) unsweetened orange juice

1.   Arrange fruit 'dippers' on a plate and sprinkle with lemon juice.
2.   Place the chocolate drops, Shape Single and orange juice in a 2 pint (1litre) bowl and microwave on Medium for 10-12 minutes until the mixture blends together, stirring twice throughout the cooking time.
3.   Serve immediately with cocktail sticks to spear fruit.

Serves 4   *300 calories per portion*

CHOCOLATE SAUCE

4 level tbsp (60ml) custard powder
2 level tbsp (30ml) cocoa
1½ pints (850ml) semi-skimmed milk
3 level tbsp (45ml) Hermesetas Sprinkle Sweet

1.   Mix the custard powder and cocoa with a little of the milk until smooth.
2.   Heat the remaining milk until almost boiling.
3.   Pour onto the custard powder, stirring all the time.
4.   Return to the pan and bring to the boil, stirring continuously. Simmer for 2 minutes.
5.   Remove from the heat and stir in the Sprinkle Sweet.

Serves 8   *75 calories per portion*

CHOCOLATE SEMOLINA

½ pint (275ml) semi-skimmed milk
2 level tbsp (15ml) semolina
1oz (25g) chocolate hazelnut spread
Hermesetas Sprinkle Sweet to taste

1. Heat the milk in a small pan nearly to boiling point.
2. Add in the semolina and cook gently for 2 minutes stirring all the time.
3. Remove from the heat and stir in the chocolate hazelnut spread and Sprinkle Sweet before serving.

Serves 2-3   *About 200 calories per portion*

MINI CHOC PUD   *(Microwave recipe)*

½oz (15g) low-fat spread
3 tsp (15ml) plain flour
Hermesetas Sprinkle Sweet
2½fl oz (65ml) milk
1oz (25g) plain chocolate drops
1 egg, size 3, separated
pinch of cream of tartar

1. Microwave the low-fat spread on High for 15 seconds.
2. Sift the flour into the low-fat spread, then add the sweetener and the milk.
3. Microwave on High for 1 minute or until thickened, stirring once.
4. Add the chocolate drops and stir until melted.
5. Beat the egg yolk into the chocolate mixture.
6. Whisk the egg white with the cream of tartar until it is stiff but not dry and fold carefully into the chocolate mixture.
7. Turn into a lightly greased dish and microwave on Defrost for 2 minutes. Serve immediately.

Serves 1   *360 calories per portion*

CHOCCY SANDWICHES AND NIBBLES

These are quick, tasty treats which need no cooking. Remember to eat them slowly, enjoying every mouthful.

- Sandwich of 2 slices wholemeal bread, 1 small sliced banana, 2 tsps (10ml) drinking chocolate. *250 calories*
- Sandwich of 2 slices slimmer's bread, toasted or plain, 1oz (25g) Cadbury's Chocolate Spread. *165 calories*
- Toasted treat of 1 slice wholemeal toast, topped with orange slices and 1 squirt Anchor Light Chocolate Mousse. *200 calories*
- Open sandwich of 1 slice wholemeal bread, topped with 2 tsps (10ml) reduced-sugar strawberry jam, 1 squirt aerosol cream, 1 sliced fun-size Mars bar. *275 calories*
- Naughty nibble of 2 crispbreads topped with 2 tsps (10ml) reduced-sugar raspberry jam, 1 Cadbury's Wispa cut in two and crumbled up. *125 calories*

THE CHOCOHOLIC'S
FOOD DIARY

All our successful Chocoholic slimmers kept a weekly Food Diary to help them stick to their diet. All you need is a notebook, divided into columns as shown overleaf. Keep it with you at all times so that you can make a note of your mood, where you were, and who you were with during each meal, snack or nibble. Once a week, analyse it yourself, using the ten pointers below.

If you feel that you have your chocoholic problem well and truly under control and don't need the diary any more, fine. However, if your weight creeps up again, or you find that your thoughts (and fingers!) are repeatedly straying towards chocolate, fill in a diary for a week, and you'll be able to nip problems in the bud before they get out of control.

POINTS TO CHECK

1. Note the time, place and mood you were in when you had difficulty in controlling choc-eating urges. Were you under pressure? Had you eaten enough during the day? Were others making your life difficult? Think about it.

2. Did you eat properly at breakfast time? If not, is there a way of making things easier – preparing your food the night before perhaps, or getting up a bit earlier? Maybe it is not as bad as it sounds and it would make tempers less frayed all round. I get up at 6.45am and enjoy a leisurely breakfast and

THE CHOCOHOLIC'S FOOD DIARY

	Monday	Tuesday	Wednesday	Thursday	Friday	Saturday	Sunday
Breakfast: Where?	Poached egg on toast At home, in kitchen standing up!						
Who with	Children, husband						
Mood	Irritable. Forced to eat, grabbing mouthfuls, family problems						
Lunch: Where?	Chicken sandwich, packet of crisps In the office						
Who with	Alone, everyone out to lunch						
Mood	Cross with myself eating crisps. Why not low-fat and fruit. Work horrendous. Fancy bar Fruit & Nut. Be good!						
Supper: Where?	Prawn tikka, boiled rice, poppadam, ½ pint lager Indian Restaurant						
Who with	Four friends						
Mood	Resisted nan bread/ fried rice. Can I last till bedtime? Fruit when I get home						
Bedtime: Where?	Ovaltine Options drink In bed						
Who with	Alone, husband watching TV!						
Mood	Good. Feel positive						

137

read the papers before starting work at 8.30am. It is worth it, honestly.

3. Did you sit down and eat your meals in a proper, civilised atmosphere? If you snatched something at a station or from a takeaway, chances are your brain didn't get a chance to register 'full' signals properly because you ate the food in such a rush. This could explain why you snacked again later in the day.

4. Is there a pattern to your snack-attacks? Does a particular person, place, TV programme trigger them? By recognising these patterns you are already half-way to curing the problem.

5. Are your meals *really* satisfying? If you have noted tummy rumblings throughout the day, it could be that you are not eating enough. Don't forget to pile on those 'free' vegetables and check that you are consuming everything you are allowed on your eating programme.

6. Are you exposing yourself to unnecessary temptation by not being prepared? Look for occasions when you went astray because you didn't have the right low-calorie snacks with you. Plan to set this right immediately. It takes only a few seconds to pop a packet of low-fat crisps and some fruit into your bag or briefcase but it could prevent you from eating several bars of chocolate later on.

7. Do you need to shop more often? It's crazy to ruin your diet because you don't have the right foods in the larder. Check if there were times when you ate something unsuitable just because there was nothing better in the house. Vow to shop more intelligently next week, adding the things you need to your list.

8. Are you leaving gaps that are too long between meals? This can happen if you are not prepared. See above!

9. Did stress or a family upset make you 'comfort eat'? If so, forgive yourself and try to deal with similar problems in a

different way next time. Don't forget that exercise is a great stress-beater.

10.   Did you do exceptionally well? Congratulate yourself and give yourself a treat immediately. If it's a choccy one, make sure it is within your daily calorie allowance and combine it with some other sensual pleasure like listening to music, or relaxing in the bath!

CALORIE GUIDE TO YOUR FAVOURITE CHOCS

On the Chocoholic Diet, you are allowed a certain amount of chocolate. Choose it from this list. For your convenience, we have divided certain popular chocolate products into calorie counted sections. These are fun-size (mostly under 100 calories), under 100 calories, 200, 250 and 300 calories.

There is also a list of chocolate biscuit products, cakes, individual chocolates, chocolate liqueurs, specialist products and even choc-erotica. Remember, watch those calories and divide larger treats up into small daily portions if you prefer. Alternatively, you can save your chocolate allowance for one or two nights but make sure it is kept out of sight in a tin until you want to nibble at it. It is better to buy your allowance daily to avoid any temptation.

CHOCOLATE *(each bar or bag)*

FUN SIZE	Calories		
Cadbury's		*Mars*	
Buttons	70	Bounty	135
Crunchie	80	Maltesers	105
Double Decker	85	Mars	80
Fudge	65	Milky Way	75
Wispa	75	Snickers	90

CALORIE GUIDE TO YOUR FAVOURITE CHOCS

Rowntree
Aero 50
Lion Bar 80
Smarties 55

Safeway
Funtime Fudge Bar 95
Funtime Honeycombe
   Bar 70
Honeycombe Crunch Bar 85

Sainsbury's
Milk Chocolate Fun Time
   Bar 105

St Michael
Crunchy bars (12 pack) 60
Fudge bars (12 pack) 90

UNDER 100 CALORIES
Cadbury's
Dairy Milk Bar (small) 95
Shoe People bar 95
Flake (99 size) 45

Nestlé
Animal Bar 100
Milkybar 65

UNDER 150 CALORIES
Cadbury's
Chomp 115
Crunchie (small) 110

Curly Wurly 130
Dairy Milk (small) 105
Fudge 130
Wildlife Bar 105

Jamesons
Oh Yes 130

Kent
Golden Crunch bar 130

Kinder
Milk Slice 125

Leaf
Lo Bar 105

Mars
Applause (5 pack) 100
Balisto 115
Bounty (5 pack) 135
Milky Way (single) 115
Twix Tea Break 140

Rowntree
Golden Cup 105
Kit Kat (2 fingers) 110

Terry's
Pryamint 135

Tobler/Suchard
Toblerone (small) 140

141

St Michael

Walnut Whip	125

UNDER 200 CALORIES

Cadbury's

Buttons (standard)	170
Creme Egg	175
Crunchie (standard)	195
Flake	170
Skippy	165
Turkish Delight	180
Fry's Turkish Delight	180
Wispa	190

Jacob / Suchard

Milka Lila Pause Corn Crisp	185

Jamesons

Ruffle bar	155
Chocolate Dip	175

Marabou

Dime bar	160

Mars

Mars (Snack Size)	180
Revels (small)	175
Ripple	155

Nestlé

Dairy Crunch	160
Milkybar	175
Milkybar Buttons	180

Rowntree

Aero (chunky)	170
Caramac (small)	165
Novo	195
Smarties (small)	175
Walnut Whip	170

St Michael

Fudge finger	180
Nutcracker	155

UNDER 250 CALORIES

Cadbury's

Bar 6	210
Caramel	245
Double Decker	235
Fruit & Nut (chunky)	245
Fry's Chocolate Cream	210
Picnic	225
Spira (2 pieces)	210
Twirl	205

Mars

Applause	220
Balisto	210
Galaxy Gold Truffle (per pack)	225
Galaxy Milk Chocolate	245
m&m's (standard)	230
Milky Way (twin)	225
Minstrels (standard)	205
Topic	230

Rowntree

Aero Mint	235
Aero Milk or Orange	230
Cabana	235
Dairy Crunch (large)	250
Kit Kat (4 finger)	245
Lion Bar	240
Milkybar (chunky)	200
Toffee Crisp	245

Safeway

Milk Chocolate Buttons	245

St Michael

Milk Chocolate with caramel	225

Terry's

Logger	245

UNDER 300 CALORIES
Cadbury's

Biscuit Boost	280
Bournville Dark	255
Buttons (large)	265
Dairy Milk (chunky)	270
Whole Nut (chunky)	270

Mars

Bounty (twin)	275
Maltesers	265
Mars (standard)	270
Twix (Twin Snacks)	280

Rowntree

Drifter	260
Munchies, Hazelnut	290
Rolo (medium)	265
Yorkie, Raisin and Biscuit	295

PER SWEET
Cadbury's

Hazel in Caramel	65
Mini Eggs	15
Wishes	80

Elizabeth Shaw

Mint Crisps	30

Ferrero Rocher 65

Rowntree

After Eight Mints	35
Rolo	25

CHOCOLATE EASTER EGGS

Easter eggs should not be eaten all in one go! Once opened and broken, they should be kept in a tin. Savour a few mouthfuls every day. The calories given include the shell and filling. Remember – measured by the 'bite', the filling is usually higher in calories than the shell which is normally made from very thin chocolate.

Cadbury's

Buttons (180g)	936
Caramel Egg (225g)	1136
Crunchie Egg (204g)	1010
Dairy Milk Heritage (220g)	1144
Flake Egg (185g)	953
Fry's Turkish Delight (220g)	979
Roses Egg (346g)	1730
Luxury Milk Tray (747g)	3735
Creme Egg (mini) (11g)	50
Creme Egg (standard) (23g)	175

Mars

Bounty (242g)	1232
m&m's (fun size)	445
Twix (212g)	1084
Maltesers Mug Egg (110g)	564
Mars Kingsize Egg (465g)	2316
Snickers (220g)	1114

Rowntree

Aero (medium)	1170
After Eight (medium)	1601
Buttons (small)	582
Dairy Box (medium)	1138
Rolo (medium)	1298
Smarties (small)	559
(medium)	1072
Quality Street (small)	612
(medium)	1145
Yorkie (medium)	1181

CHOC-EROTICA
Spencer and Fleetwood

Naughty Bits selection (*calories per individual chocolate*):

Drunken Bum	59
Nipple	81
Belgian Chocolate Willie (90g of solid chocolate)	540
Boob (90g of solid chocolate)	540
Cream Filled Willie (100g)	684

CHOCOLATE BISCUITS
(per biscuit)
Asda

Chocolate Digestive (plain or milk)	80
Oat Round (plain or milk)	85
Take a Break Milk Chocolate Fruit and Nut Bar	95

Take a Break Milk Chocolate
  Muesli Bar   95

Burton's
Chocolate Chip & Hazelnut
  Cookie   55
Chocolate Chip Cookie   55
Jaffa Cake   40
Milk Chocolate Snapjack   85
Plain Chocolate Fruit
  Snapjack   90
Viscount, Mint or Orange   90
Wagon Wheel   170

Cadbury's
Bar 6   210
Bournville Digestive   45
Bournville Sandwich   120
Dairy Milk Sandwich   120
Milk Chocolate Digestive   45
Chocolate Orange
  Digestive   45

Crawford's
Choc Chip & Hazelnut
  Cookie   40
Choc Chip & Orange
  Cookie   40
Pennywise Bourbon
  Cream   60
Pennywise Chocolate Chip
  Oatie   35

Fox's
Chocolate Orange Cream   75
Choc Chip Cream   65
Natural Crunch, Choc Chip
  & Almond Original Choc
  Chip Cookie   80

Gateway
Bourbon   65
Choc 'n Nut Cookie   50
Chocolate Wheatmeal –
  Milk or Plain   65
Milk Chocolate Orange
  Sandwich   125
Milk Chocolate
  Sandwich   125
Milk Chocolate Shortcake   95

Huntley & Palmer
Chocolate Digestive, Milk
  or Plain   65
Choc Chip 'n Nut Cookie   45
Double Choc Chip Cookie   80

Jacob's
Club – Coffee, Fruit, Milk,
  Mint, Orange, Lemon
  and Lime   115
Club, Plain   110
Trio   125

Lyon's
Maryland Cookies –
Choc Chip, Choc Chip &

Hazelnut, Chocolate &
Chocolate Chip,
Traditional Chocolate
Chip   50

Macdonalds
Taxi	80
Yo Yo – Mint, Orange	100
Yo Yo – Toffee	95

McVitie's
Bandit or Boaster	95
Chocolate Biscuit Finger, Milk or Plain	25
Chocolate Hob-Nob, Milk or Plain	80
Chocolate Homewheat, Milk or Plain	85
54321	110
Jaffa Cake	45
Gold	130
Hob-Nob bar	160
Penguin	125
Solar Choc Chip	110

Peak Freans
Bourbon	60
Coated Mallow, Milk or Orange	55
Snowball	130

Safeway
Bourbon Cream	70

Butter Chocolate Chip Shortcake	100
Chocolate Cream	65
Chocolate Digestive, Milk or Plain	65
Chocolate Orange Crunch Cream	60
Chocolate Nut Cookie	55
Milk Chocolate Caramel Shortcake	95
Milk Chocolate Caramel Wafer	85
Milk Chocolate Coronet Cream	90
Milk Chocolate Digestive Bar	95
Milk Chocolate Finger	45
Milk Chocolate Fruit & Nut bar	95
Milk Chocolate Orange Finger Wafer	40
Milk Chocolate Orange Sandwich	135
Milk Chocolate Sandwich	125
Milk Chocolate Shortcake	105
Milk Chocolate Sunata or Orange Cream	60
Milk Chocolate Teacake	50
Plain Chocolate Finger	50
Snowball	60

Sainsbury's

All Butter Chocolate Choc Chip Cookie	100
Bourbon Cream	60
Chocolate Chip Nibble Cookie	15
Choc Chip Oat & Coconut Crunch	35
Choc Chip Shortbread Ring	65
Chocolate & Nut Cookie	50
Chocolate Digestive, Milk or Plain	75
Chocolate Finger, Milk or Plain	25
Chocolate Rustic, Milk or Plain	75
Chocolate Wafer, Milk or Plain	45
Italian Cocoa Cream Cookie	95
Jaffa Cake	45
Milk Chocolate Crunch Bar	135
Milk Chocolate Crunch, half-coated	35
Milk Chocolate Nice	50
Milk Chocolate Petit Beurre	50
Milk Chocolate Rich Tea	60
Mini Oat & Chocolate Cookie	15
Plain Chocolate Ginger Biscuit	60
Plain Chocolate Ginger Crunch, half-coated	35
Plain Chocolate Orange Biscuit	60
Snowball	105
Viva, Mint/Plain, Chocolate/Milk	145
Viva, Orange/Plain, Vanilla/Milk	140

St Michael

Bourbon	65
Chocolate & Black Cherry Sponge Thin	55
Chocolate Chip Cookie	60
Chocolate Chip & Hazelnut Cookie	55
Milk Chocolate Crunch	35
Jaffa Cake	45
Milk Chocolate Caramel Wafer	95
Milk Chocolate Currant Topped Wafer	120
Milk Chocolate Digestive Biscuit	65
Milk Chocolate Wafer Finger	45
Milk Chocolate Oat Crunchie	75
Milk Chocolate Orange Sandwich Bar	130
Milk Chocolate Tea Cake	80
Plain Chocolate Digestive	65

Plain Chocolate Ginger
Biscuit 45
Plain Chocolate Mint
Sandwich Bar 110
Plain Chocolate Oat
Crunchie 80
Traditional Choc Chip
Cookie 80
Viennese Chocolate
Sandwich 75

Tesco
Bourbon Cream 65
Chocolate Wafer 80
Chocolate Digestive, Milk
or Plain 85
Economy Chocolate Chip
Cookie 55
Economy Milk Chocolate
Digestive 65
Jaffa Cake 40
Milk Chocolate Teacake 60
Milk Chocolate Orange
Sandwich 120
Milk Chocolate
Sandwich 125
Milk Chocolate Coated
Digestive Bar 95
Milk Chocolate Shortcake
Bar 96

Waitrose
Bourbon 60
Chocolate Nut Cookie 50

Chocolate Chip Cookie
(mini) 15
Chocolate Chip Orange
Flavour Cookie 50
Chocolate Chip
Shortbread 100
Chocolate Ginger Crunch 30
Chocolate Petit Beurre,
Milk or Plain 50
Chocolate Wafer Finger 45
Milk Chocolate Digestive 65

Walkers
Chocolate Chip
Shortbread Ring 70
Chocolate Chip
Shortbread 70
Chocolate Ring (coated) 65

CHOCOLATE BREAKFAST CEREALS
(per 1oz/28g)

Cereal Partners
Coca Shreddies 101

Co-op
Choc Chip Muesli 114

Deeside
Choc Chip Muesli 114

Kellogg's
Coco Pops	108

Lyons Tetley
Coco Brek	101

Prewetts
Choco Muesli	105

Sainsbury's
Coco Snaps	98

St Michael
Chocolate flake Crunchy Muesli	125

Tesco
Coco Puffs	100

Weetabix
Weetos	94

CHOCOLATE CAKES *(per cake unless otherwise stated)*

Asda
Milk Chocolate Jaffa Ripple	85
Milk Chocolate Junior Roll	120
Milk Chocolate and Mint Junior Roll	120

Cadbury's
Chocolate Cake *(per 1oz/28g)*	111
Chocolate Whips *(per 1oz/28g)*	120
Coconut Topper	65
Flake Cake	120
Fudge Diamond	110
Mini Roll	115
Jam Mini Roll	95
Mini Logs *(per 1oz/28g)*	118
Swiss Gâteau	1075

Dunkin Donuts
Chocolate Chip Cookie	130
Chocolate Frosted Yeast Ring	245

Gateway
Maitre D' (per 1oz/28g)
Black Forest Cake	68
Black Forest Gateau	91
Chocolate Dairy Cream Sponge	82
Double Chocolate and Walnut Gateau	91
Illegal Chocolate Cake (Louisiana)	102

Iceland
Chocolate & Grand Marnier Gateau	2520
Chocolate Flavour Sponge	610

Doughnut with Chocolate
Icing   225
Doughnut with Chocolate
Orange Filling   285
Doughnut with Chocolate
Vermicelli   220
Raspberry and Chocolate
Torte   1295

Lyons
Small cakes
Caramel Chocolate Roll   110
Chocolate Cup Cake   130
Chocolate Fancy   120
Chocolate Slice   110
Large cakes
Chocolate Sandwich   855
Chocolate Super Roll   825
Chocolate and Vanilla
Swiss Roll   825

McVities (per 1oz/28g)
Chocolate Cake   105
Frozen cakes
Black Forest Cake   90
Black Forest Cheesecake   93
Black Forest Gateau   81
Black Forest Party
Gateau   85
Chocolate and Cherry
Gateau   82
Chocolate Meringue
Gateau   108
Double Chocolate Gateau   95

Double Chocolate Party
Gateau   98

Mr Kipling (per 1oz/28g)
Chocolate Viennese
Shell   133
Chocolate Sponge   102

Safeway
Small cakes
Chocolate mini roll   125
Large cakes
Chocolate and
Blackcurrant Gateau   965
Chocolate Chip Cake   1430
Chocolate Log with
Buttercream   1765
Chocolate Sponge
Sandwich   880

Sainsbury's
Small cakes
Chocolate Cup Cake   130
Chocolate & Orange
Bakewell   210
Chocolate Delight   119
Chocolate Viennese
Fancy   155
Mini Chocolate Swiss
Roll   115
Large cakes
Chocolate Decorated
Sandwich   106

Chocolate Flavour Swiss
Roll 105
Chocolate Orange Swiss
Roll 102
Chocolate Sponge with
Jaffa Orange & Vanilla
Buttercream 930
Milk Chocolate Roll 109

St Michael
Small cakes
Chocolate Covered Mini
Roll 145
Chocolate Cup Cake 135
Fresh Cream Chocolate
Eclair 155
Meringue with Chocolate
Cream 175
Big cakes
Chocolate Fudge Brownies
(per 1oz/28g) 125
Sponge Gateau with
Chocolate Butter-
cream 990
Frozen cakes
Black Forest Gateau 1540
Chocolate Layer Cake
Gateau 2650
Swiss rolls (per 1oz/28g)
Chocolate Covered
Sponge Roll 820
Chocolate Sponge Roll
with Chocolate
Buttercream 112

Tesco
Small cakes
Chocolate Orange Roll 120
Large cakes
Chocolate Bar Gâteau *(per
1oz/28g)* 90
Chocolate Orange
Marble Cake 1015
Chocolate Sponge
Sandwich 715
Fresh Cream Chocolate
Sponge Bar *(per 1oz/
28g)* 91

Waitrose
Large cakes (per 1oz/28g)
Chocolate Gâteau Roule,
Black Cherry 102
Chocolate Gâteau Roule,
Buttercream 118
Chocolate Sandwich 130
Milk Chocolate Covered
Roll 121

CHOCOLATE DRINKS

Alcoholic
(1/6 gill/pub measure)

Cadbury's Chocolate Cream
Liqueur 75

151

CALORIE GUIDE TO YOUR FAVOURITE CHOCS

Beverages

Associated Dairies
Flavoured Long Life Milk
(per 1 pint/568ml):
Chocolate   405

Breaktime Flavoured Milks
Chocolate (200ml
  carton)   140
Chocolate (500ml
  bottle)   355

Cadbury's *(per 1oz/28g)*
Bournvita Malted
  Chocolate Drink   105
Chocolate Break, milk
  chocolate drink   105
Chocolate Break, plain
  chocolate drink   105
Chocolate Milk
  (per 180ml carton)   185
Chocolate Milk
  (per 480ml carton)   445
Drinking Chocolate *(per
  serving)*   65

Dairy Crest
Chocolate Flite *(per 200ml
  carton)*   125

Express Dairies
Stripes Flavoured Milk,
  Chocolate *(per

17.6 fl oz/500ml)   305
Munch Bunch Milk Shakes,
  Chocolate *(per 180g)*   135

Mars
Mars Milk Drink *(per 200ml
  carton)*   200

Sainsbury's
Low Fat Flavoured Milk,
  Chocolate *(per 500ml
  carton)*   300

St Ivel
Crazy Milk, Chocolate *(per
  200ml carton)*   125

St Michael
Chocolate Milkshake *(per
  6.4 fl oz/180ml)*   155
Chocolate Semi-Skimmed
  Milk Drink *(per
  1 fl oz/28ml)*   19

Scottish Pride
Chocolate Flavoured Milk
  (per 200ml carton)   140

Tesco
Chocolate Milkshake *(per
  200ml carton)*   120

Waitrose

Chocolate Milkshake *(per 180ml carton)* 155

CHOCOLATE ICECREAM

Iceland Cornish Choc Ice 125

Iceland Cornish Choc Ice (6 pack) 115

Iceland Mint Choc Ice (8 pack) 100

Loseley Montezuma Choc *(per individual pot)* 110

Lyons Maid Dark Ice Choc Ice 125

Lyons Maid King Cone Choc Ice 200

Mars Icecream 220

Ross Choc Ice 130

Ross Chocolog 130

Ross Chocolog – Strawberry 110

Tesco Choc Ice 130

Tesco Choc Nut Icecream Cone 215

Tesco Choc Nut Lolly 120

Walls Bonanza 200

Walls Chunky Choc Ice 165

Walls Feast 255

Walls Choc and Nut Cup 170

COUNSELLING GROUPS

If you feel that you need expert help to control your chocoholism or any other form of eating disorder, don't hesitate to seek it. In the first instance, you should consult your GP. The groups below are also very helpful. Do enclose a stamped, addressed envelope with your enquiry.

The Eating Disorders
    Association
c/o The Priory Centre
11 Priory Road
High Wycombe
Bucks
HP13 6SL
Tel: 0494 521431
(11.30am – 2.30pm)
and
Sackville Place
44/48 Magdalen Street
Norwich
Norfolk
NR3 1JE
Tel: 0603 621414
(9.00am – 4.00pm)

BANISH (Bulimia and
    Anorexia Nervosa
    Intermediate Self Help)
27 Lawrence Avenue
Lytham St Anne's
Lancashire
FY8 3LG

The Maisner Centre for
    Eating Disorders
PO Box 464
Hove
East Sussex
BN3 2BN
Tel: 0273 729818

Society for Primary Cause
    Analysis by Hypnosis
13 Beechwood Road
Sanderstead
Croydon
Surrey
(write to The President)
Tel: 081-657 3624

If you would like to write to
    me, my address is:
Sally Ann Voak
PO Box 618
Coulsdon
Surrey
CR5 1RU